"This is one of the most powerful books I've read. Every chapter, every word has stuck with me. Pete's honesty and openness captivated me. As I read the first half of the book—on living with Parkinson's—I laughed hysterically at Chapter 8, 'What's So Funny?' I sang aloud in Chapter 10, 'My Parkinson's Friends.' Chapter 12, 'How You Can Help,' should be part of APDA's staff training. Chapter 14, 'The Evolution of a P-Man,' gave me insight to the emotional stages people with Parkinson's go through as their disease progresses. I sobbed at times as I read the second half of the book—on dying with Parkinson's. Pete brings up issues that we all need to discuss, but we avoid them because dying seems so frightening. Pete's book brings a fresh perspective by showing how much we have to be grateful for and how much control we have as we learn to live and die with Parkinson's."
—Jean Allenbach, Executive Director, Northwest Chapter of the American Parkinson's Disease Association (APDA)

"Pete's book on living and dying with Parkinson's disease is one of the best I've read—about any debilitating illness. Once I began reading, I could not put it down. The book is engaging, insightful, humorous, and wise. It is filled with illuminating personal examples and meaningful stories. Pete's writing is extremely clear and intelligent. His story may be sad—as illness and grief legitimately are—but it is not morose. In fact, this book is eloquent and triumphal. I want everyone I know with Parkinson's disease, along with those who are living with other terminal illnesses, to read this book."
—Trudy James, chaplain and film producer of *Speaking of Dying*

"Pete's honest and courageous story is full of loving guidance for all of us who are alive, knowing that we are all living into our

dying. Regardless of where you are on your life journey, you will explore possibilities about end-of-life choices that affect you and your loved ones. Pete demonstrates how the fear of death is greatly diminished when we plan, as best we can, with honesty and love."
—Phyllis Shacter, author of *Choosing to Die, A Personal Story: Elective Death by Voluntarily Stopping Eating and Drinking (VSED) in the Face of Degenerative Disease*

"In the field of Aging, an increasing number of uncomfortable 'D' words confront many of us: Disease, Disability, Denial, Depression, Dying, Death. They are the realities that both face us and scare us as we age. Pete's lucid book doesn't shy away from mentioning them, but he tempers his story with additional concepts such as Discovery and Delight. His book offers wisdom and wit to people living with Parkinson's disease. His honesty and sense of generosity and gratitude reveal a man with courage and an ongoing commitment to the value of communication and connection.
This book will inform and inspire others and answer many of the questions people have about what it is like to live—and eventually die—with a debilitating and incurable disease."
—Rebecca Crichton, Executive Director, Northwest Center for Creative Aging

"If you are you squeamish, fearful, or embarrassed about having Parkinson's or being near someone with the disease, this slender book, this refreshingly honest, no-holds-barred overview is a must-read. It is crisp, direct, kind, informational, loving, and occasionally humorous. The perfect guide for people with Parkinson's, their families, and their friends."
—Griggs Irving, retired educator, PwP

"For all its lightness of tone, I found the book quite moving. Even though neither I nor anyone I know has Parkinson's, I feel inspired to be a better person after having read it."
—Gary A. Kass, University of Missouri Press

"Pete's wisdom, research, and gentle humor illuminate this

personal story of living with Parkinson's disease, including the rarely discussed late stages. Pete has written a candid, unflinching account of his decisions about how he wants to live and die with this disease. Family members of people with the disease will benefit from his thoughtful insights. This well-written book is a timely addition to the Parkinson's bookshelf."
—Carin Mack, MSW, ACSW, Geriatric Health Consultant

"This book will resonate with everyone in the Parkinson's universe—its victims, their loved ones, and their caregivers. But not them alone. Anyone—even those not currently facing their own mortality—can benefit from Parkinson Pete's knowledge and wisdom, conveyed with genial humor. Here's proof that a book about dying the good death can be instructive, heart-warming, and entertaining."
—Catherine Treadgold, writer and editor

"What does it mean to live a good life with Parkinson's? Pete shares his journey from diagnosis to late-stage Parkinson's. His humor, experience, and research combine for an entertaining and illuminating read. Pete empowers his readers to live a good life with Parkinson's, while also insisting that they lay the groundwork for what will be a good death with Parkinson's."
—Heather Danso, GCFP, E-YRT

Parkinson Pete on Living and Dying with Parkinson's Disease

PETER G. BEIDLER

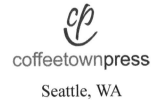

coffeetownpress

Seattle, WA

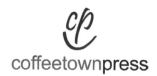

coffeetownpress

Epicenter Press
6524 NE 181st St.
Suite 2
Kenmore, WA 98028

www.epicenterpress.com
www.coffeetownpress.com

This memoir is a truthful recollection of actual events in the author's life, augmented by his reading of the wise words of others. Some conversations have been recreated or supplemented. The names and details of some individuals have been changed to respect their privacy. The medical information in this book is true and complete to the best of the author's knowledge. Any advice or recommendations, especially those related to medical, legal, or financial issues, are made without guarantee on the part of the author or publisher. This book is not a substitute for professional advice. Every situation is different.

Cover design by Sabrina Sun
Back-cover portrait by Bill Curr

Parkinson Pete on Living and Dying with Parkinson's Disease
Copyright © 2020 by Peter G. Beidler

ISBN: 9781603815628 (Trade Paper)
ISBN: 9781603815635 (eBook)

Library of Congress Control Number: 2019951674

Produced in the United States of America

For Anne

You are the best person I've ever known.
You are the maker of good things to eat,
the provider of good things to do,
the nurturer of near-perfect children
and absolutely perfect grandchildren.
Thank you for being at my side for this
tumultuous half-century and more.
You are a gentlewoman and gentle woman.
You are a woman of strength, compassion, grace
and good sense. You embody all of the
possibilities of love.
I thank you and I love you.

Contents

Part Two: Dying with Parkinson's Disease

Acknowledgments

I AM GRATEFUL TO MY WIFE ANNE, my children, Paul, Kurt, Calloway, and Nora, and my nine grandchildren for their cheerful forbearance in these past fifteen years as I adjusted to the shifting sands of my Parkinson's; to the many members of my Parkinson's medical and physical therapy teams for their patience and wisdom; to my Seattle Parkinson's friends for their cheerful perseverance despite the limitations that our disease imposes on us; to Jim and Mary Phillips for their good-humored support for many years; to Griggs Irving, Fran Miller, Elli Fox, Catherine Treadgold, Rebecca Crichton, Trudy James, Peter Lynch, Heather Danso, Carin Mack, and BetteJane Camp, for their corrections to early drafts; and to Marion Egge for her lifetime of devoted editorial assistance.

Preface: Walking the Parkinson's Trail

THOSE OF US WHO HAVE PARKINSON'S DISEASE spend our last decade or two (or sometimes even three) learning about our disease. Some of us—like me—are arrogant enough to think that what we have learned may help others. I spent my professional life as a teacher of English and American literature at Lehigh University. Now, as I approach the end of my life, it seems natural to want to leave behind some signposts to mark the Parkinson's trail for those who come after.

One of the pleasures of my early days in Seattle was walking. I walked to the post office, to the bank, to the gym, to the Ballard and the Greenwood branch libraries, to the bus stop so I could go south to the architecturally stunning Seattle Public Library or east to the University of Washington's Suzallo Library, to several senior centers, to the Ballard Health Club for exercise, to Northwest Hospital for yoga, and so on. There were a lot of steps on my Parkinson's trail.

I am honored to present here, at the start of my book, "Walking," a poem my dear wife Anne wrote for me and my Parkinson's friends back in 2010, when I was still able to do a lot of walking:

Walking
by Anne E. Beidler

Your left foot drags,
Your right foot trips on a tuft of grass,
But you keep on walking.

Your hand shakes
When you try to count your pills,
But you keep on counting.

You try so hard to speak clearly.
Sometimes people can't hear you,
But you keep on talking.

If I had to deal with all the surprises of Parkinson's,
I would probably just sit on the sofa all day
And watch TV,
And complain about the TV,
And complain about the weather,
And complain about Parkinson's.

But you don't.
You keep moving.
Yoga, dance, and walking, walking, walking.
Singing, bicycling, and walking, walking, walking.
Working out in the gym, working down in your workshop,
And walking, walking, walking.

I cannot walk so much now, in 2019. My feet freeze, my legs buckle, I fall forward, I bang up my knees. My wrists and my shoulders are sore from catching myself as I careen into walls and floors. I don't go out now without a walker. It is almost impossible for me to cross a street because I know that I will probably freeze partway across. It is almost impossible for me to get on and off the wonderful Metro buses of Seattle. Anne now drives me to most of the places I need to go to, so I don't go as many places, or as often, as I used to. My Parkinson's trail has gotten narrower and shorter than it used to be, but it is a wonderful trail, and I feel fortunate to have walked on it as long and as far as I have, and to have met so many fine fellow travelers.

I started writing this book to help me understand the disease that has so dominated my life for the past decade. It occurred to me that what I have written may also be of interest to my current and future fellow travelers—the men and women who share or will share my diagnosis—and to members of their families.

A few of the shorter chapters—6, 7, 9, and 14—have been published before. The rest are presented here for the first time. My intended audience for **Part One: Living with Parkinson's Disease** is people newly or recently diagnosed—and people who want to understand enough about the disease that they can help a family member or friend who has been diagnosed. My intended audience for **Part Two: Dying with Parkinson's Disease** is people who are approaching the later stages—and their families. The overall message of both parts is the same: a) Parkinson's is different for everyone; b) Parkinson's is not as bad as you think it will be; c) there is much that you can do to improve your life; and, most important; d) you need to take charge. This book is designed especially to let people whose lives have been touched by Parkinson's know that they have a large measure of control over their disease. They absolutely do not need to sit meekly back and watch Parkinson's ruin their lives and then take their lives. They can—indeed, they must— take charge of both their living with Parkinson's and their dying with it.

There is a certain chrono-logic to the order of the chapters: they move generally from diagnosis to death, but each chapter is more or less self-contained. The chapters can be read in any order, depending on the interests of particular readers. Those who read through the book from front to back may notice that I repeat some ideas in more than one chapter. I could apologize for that, but I don't. Every teacher knows that repetition can sometimes make a point more memorable and emphatic.

Note: This is my second "Parkinson Pete" book. The first, *Parkinson Pete's Bookshelves: Reviews of Eighty-Nine Books about Parkinson's Disease* (Seattle: Coffeetown Press, 2018), was almost entirely about what other men and women—doctors, patients, novelists—had to say about Parkinson's disease. This book, on the other hand, is based almost entirely on my own experiences. I occasionally refer to one or more of the eighty-nine books referenced in the original Parkinson Pete book. To save space I usually give only the author and the page number. You will find the full reference in a list of works cited at the end of this book, as well as the reference number of such books as they are given in *Parkinson Pete's Bookshelves*: A23, B19, C4, etc.

Part One:

Living with
Parkinson's Disease

1. Becoming Parkinson Pete

AT THE START I WAS ASHAMED of my disease. I wondered what I had done wrong to bring it on. I wanted no one to know about it. Then, as people found out, I was annoyed to discover that so many people knew so little about this disease that was slowly taking over my life. Then, it annoyed me to discover that people who knew me seemed to see in me only my Parkinson's. I knew there was a whole lot more to Pete than Pete's tremors, Pete's soft voice, Pete's slowness, Pete's stutters and stumbles and falls. It annoyed me to discover that people thought of me as "that man with Parkinson's (his name is Pete)" rather than as "that man named Pete (he has Parkinson's)." I was Pete first; the Parkinson's was just a footnote to the main text.

At the start I quite agreed with the men and women with this disease who insisted that they were not their disease and their disease was not them. I didn't like it when people saw me as little more than an old man disabled by his Parkinson's. Disabled? Not hardly! I was not unable to walk; I just walked with a shuffle and sometimes I stumbled. I was not unable to talk; I just talked softly, slurred some words, and sometimes stuttered. I was not unable to dress myself; it just took longer, and buttons were a bitch. I was not unable to feed myself; I just dropped some forkfuls of salad, found gravy stains on my shirt, and sometimes had a little difficulty swallowing. I was not unable to type; I just typed slowly, made lots and lots of mistakes, and sometimes, reading back over what I had just typed, had no idea what I had meant to say. But I was not disabled, not an invalid; I was still in most ways as abled and as valid as ever.

As the disease matured in me, however, and I matured in the disease, I have grown to see that, indeed, I now pretty much *am* my Parkinson's. My disease determines how I sleep, what time I get up, what I wear, when, what, how, and how much I eat, how much food I spill, and whether I can safely help set and clear the table. My disease determines where I go, how I get there, which stairways I use, whether I can risk going out without my walker, who I visit, for how long, and whether I can carry my own suitcase, whether I can go to a play or a movie, where I sit in a theater, which restaurants I go to, what kinds of carpentry projects I can safely work on, whether I can answer the phone when it rings, whether I can get to the front door in time when the doorbell rings, what books I read, what I write about, how I think about end-of-life issues, and so forth.

As my disease has come front-and-center, I am no longer ashamed of my Parkinson's, nor do I try to deny or conceal it. The term "disabled" no longer drives me crazy. It is better than other terms, such as "crippled," "retarded," "village idiot," "good for nothing," "useless," "helpless," "hopeless." I don't drive anymore, but my Parkinson's gets me a blue "Disabled" parking tag that I can hang from the mirror when Anne drives me some place I need to be.

The title of Stephen Crane's 1895 novel *The Red Badge of Courage* refers to the wound that proved its wearer was a brave warrior who did not run away from a battle. I have come to think of my bright blue "Disabled" parking tag as a kind of blue badge of courage. Living with this neurodegenerative disease and noticing that it relentlessly robs me of one ability after another requires and inspires and invites courage. People with Parkinson's deserve a badge, and I wear my blue mirror tag with a certain smug pride.

I resist thinking of Parkinson's as a fight to be fought, but if having Parkinson's is a fight, it is not a fair one. It is a heavyweight pro fighting a welterweight novice. The advantage is all on the side of the disease. Parkinson's always wins. Perhaps the only way to beat Parkinson's is to cheat it of its final triumph by dying of something else first.

We people with Parkinson's are a courageous lot. We find ways to grow into our disease, to accept it knowing that we will almost certainly someday be knocked down by it. We learn to embrace our disease. We learn to exhibit what another American novelist, Ernest Hemingway, called courage. In a letter to Scott Fitzgerald in 1926, Hemingway defined courage as "grace under pressure." Parkinson's keeps the pressure on us by robbing us of one element of independence after another. We can best deal with that pressure by showing grace, which might be defined as elegant calmness or dignified acceptance.

More and more insistently, my disease has become the controlling influence in my life and the generator of my thoughts about life and death.

Living with Parkinson's disease has helped me to see how little autonomy I still have, but also how much autonomy I still have, even as the disease relentlessly robs me of the power to resist its steady advance. Dying with Parkinson's disease has helped me realize I am still the boss.

I am writing this book in part to show others that they can both live well and die well with Parkinson's. Even as they lose round after round to the heavyweight pro, they can, by exhibiting courage and grace, remain the boss.

2. My Diagnosis

Early in 2004, when I was sixty-four, I initiated discussions with the administration at Lehigh University leading to my retirement a year-and-a-half later. That spring I contracted Lyme disease and was put on a heavy dose of antibiotics. On a warm day in the fall of that year, my wife Anne and I went to an afternoon movie. The theater was air-conditioned and I was wearing a short-sleeved shirt. I sat to Anne's right. We were holding hands, my left hand in her right hand. We both felt a strange shivering or quivering in my left forearm. She later described it this way: "It felt like a snake slithering up inside his left arm."

A couple of months later, partway through the fall semester, I began to notice that my left hand sometimes shook a little when I was teaching. I noticed it especially when I held a book in that hand or papers to distribute to my students. I reluctantly decided that I should go see my family doctor. I knew a little about Parkinson's because Jo, my older sister, had the disease. But surely I did not have that disease. No, no. I had seen my sister suffer with Parkinson's—the shaking, the stumbling, the constipation, the slow but inexorable reduction in her ability to move, the nausea resulting from the medications she took to try—with limited success—to minimize the symptoms. On a Fourth of July picnic in 2005, my sister fell down four times. I wanted no part of her disease.

My family doctor was puzzled by my slight left-hand tremor. "It might be several things, Pete," he said, "or nothing at all. Let's run some tests to rule out some possibilities. I remember that last spring you had a touch of Lyme disease. The antibiotics we put you on knocked that out, but we'll run a blood test to make sure it hasn't come back. And let's do a brain MRI to make sure you don't have a tumor cooking in there. You're not claustrophobic, are you?"

I wasn't.

When the Lyme analysis came back negative, the doctor scheduled an MRI. I entered the narrow tube almost hoping I had a brain tumor. I wanted a quick affliction, not the slow but inevitable deterioration that was called Parkinson's. But it was not a brain tumor. *Sigh.*

After several months of wondering why my left arm had a tremor, my family doctor, perhaps suspecting that I had Parkinson's—though he never spoke the word—sent me to a movement disorder specialist at the University of Pennsylvania Hospital in Philadelphia, seventy-five miles from home. Anne and I drove down for our appointment.

Parking near the university was a challenge. We finally found a small lot with an attendant.

"It's a hot day," I said to the attendant. "Is it okay if we park over there in that shady spot?"

"No. Shade spot is reserved. Park in sun." He pointed.

"That's ominous," I told Anne as I pulled into the sunny spot.

We walked the few blocks to the hospital. The movement disorder specialist was a pleasant-enough middle-aged woman. She asked me some questions and then had me perform simple movements—tapping my thumb and forefinger, touching my nose with my eyes closed, walking down the corridor and back, seeing if I could keep my balance when she jerked my shoulders back, and so on.

Then she asked me to take off my sneakers. I thought she wanted to examine my feet, but it was my sneakers she wanted to see. She turned them over and looked at the soles.

"I noticed that you dragged or scuffled your left foot when you walked," she said, "and your shoes confirm that. See, the left sneaker is worn down way more than the right one."

"I had noticed that my left foot flopped down differently," I said, "but I never thought to look at the bottoms of my sneaks. So what does that tell us?"

"It tells us—along with other evidence—that you most likely have Parkinson's disease." She went on to tell us that there were no imaging or chemical tests to diagnose the disease, only the physical evidence itself—the tremors, the non-symmetrical attack on one side first, the irregular walking, the decreased arm swing when I walked.

"How much do you know about Parkinson's?" she asked me.

"Too much," I said. "My sister has Parkinson's. But I didn't know it was contagious or hereditary."

"It is not contagious, and it is not exactly hereditary, though many people with the disease also have a relative or two who had or have the disease. They say that heredity loads the gun but environment pulls the trigger."

"What does that mean? What gun?"

"No gun, really. It just means that some people in your family may have a genetic predisposition to get Parkinson's, but something in the environment gives you the disease. Where did you and your sister grow up?"

"Eastern Pennsylvania, sixty miles north of here."

"City or country?"

"Country."

"Were your parents farmers?"

"No. My father was an architect. But we lived in the country."

"Then you and your sister grew up drinking well water?"

"Spring water, actually. What about it?"

"My best guess is that the local farmers up there used pesticides and herbicides on their fields, and that trace amounts of those harsh chemicals percolated down into the ground water that you and your sister drank. I am sorry to have to be the one to tell you this news, but at least now you have a name for it, and we can begin to treat it."

"Treat it? My sister is taking—I don't know what she is taking—but it doesn't help much. What do you mean by 'treat' it?"

"Well, I assume you know that there is no known cure for Parkinson's, though medical researchers are working on several possible avenues of inquiry that may lead to a cure, possibly fairly soon. Meanwhile, there are medicines that seem to slow down the progression of the disease and that give relief—for a while—from some of the symptoms. And there is growing evidence that getting lots of exercise helps."

"My sister takes little yellow pills. They nauseate her."

"Those are probably dopamine pills. People with Parkinson's have brains that for some reason make less and less dopamine. It is a slow process. By the time the physical symptoms become evident, your brain is making only about a quarter of the dopamine it used to make. The dopamine is what gives you the ability to move. The pills are a kind of artificial or synthetic dopamine that let you continue moving."

"When do I start?"

"On the pills? Not for a while. No rush. Your symptoms are minimal. But you can start on the exercise. Walk. Take out a membership in a gym. Work out. Be active. The yellow pills can wait until you really need them."

"Well, thanks," I said. "Okay, I guess we got what we came for. Anne, do you have any questions?"

"Is there anything I can do?" Anne asked.

"Take care of yourself. Both of you can start on your bucket lists. How long have you two been married?"

"Forty-three years," Anne replied. "Peter is going to retire at the end of this year, and then we'll be moving to Seattle."

"Seattle. What takes you there? I don't think too many people think of Seattle as a retirement destination."

"Not too many people have three of their four children and half of their grandkids living there," Anne said. "But it sounds like Peter will need a neurologist. Can you recommend anyone in Seattle?"

"I'll give you a list. There is a lot of research on Parkinson's going on out there, so you'll be in good hands. Hold on while I make a copy of a couple of pages from a national directory of movement disorder specialists."

We held on, in utter silence, until she came back with the list.

"Here are some names from Seattle and Bellevue—which I guess is a city just across some big lake from Seattle. I don't know any of these people personally, but there are lots to choose from. There are even a couple of Parkinson's research centers."

"Thanks, Doctor," I said, forcing a smile. "You've been a big help." That was a lie, of course. She had been no help at all. All she had done was confirm my worst fears and dash my hopes for a fun and productive retirement. "Well, I guess we had better head on back before the afternoon rush hour starts."

"I am sorry I don't have better news for you," she said. "But actually, the news is not all bad. There are way worse things you could have. You'll find that there are several effective medications that can help you when the disease progresses a little further, and there are even some surgical options. Meanwhile, you can go to a physical therapist up your way and get started on exercise routines. You are going to live a good long time."

"Okay," I said, but I was not at all sure I wanted to live a good long time with this stupid disease. "Again, thanks." We shook hands. Then Anne and I left.

I couldn't wait to get out of there. We walked back to the park-in-sun lot and retrieved our hot car.

"I'll drive," Anne said. "You've got a lot to think about."

"Whatever."

I had tried to put on a brave front there in the doctor's office, but actually I was angry, sad, disappointed, and worried. Mostly just angry at the unfairness of it all. After forty years of teaching I was finally going to be my own man. But now I was going to have to live out my life as a dependent invalid. And poor Anne, after more than forty years of raising a husband and four kids, she was going to have to spend her so-called golden years taking care of that dependent invalid. What was fair about any of that?

When we got to Willow Grove—about halfway home—I asked Anne to pull over and let me out.

"What? Why? There will be a restaurant up ahead where you can use a toilet."

"I don't want to use a toilet. Just pull over. Now, please." She did. I got out.

"Are you going to throw up?"

"No. I just want to be alone. I'm going to walk home. The good doctor said to get exercise so I might as well get started. You go on." I slammed the door and started walking. She pulled out and drove on without me.

I found her in the parking lot of a Howard Johnson's about two miles ahead. She came out to meet me.

"I'm sorry about the diagnosis," she said. "I'll walk home with you. We can come down tomorrow in the Suburban and get the car."

"You're nuts," I said. "Home is thirty miles. Don't be silly."

"That was Plan A. If you'd rather, Plan B is we go in and have a cup of soup, use the toilets, and then drive on home. I have a couple of steaks you can broil on the charcoal grill tonight."

"What kind of soup they got?"

"Cream of celery and Manhattan clam chowder. I thought maybe the Manhattan clam. I heard that out west they have only the New England style cream-based chowder."

"Plan B it is, then," I said. "Be a shame to let those steaks go to waste. Besides, I am not sure this worn left sneaker will make it home if I walk the whole way. I should have brought my hiking boots. Let's go get a cup of Plan B."

"Good," she said. "I didn't much like Plan A."

3. An Incurable Teacher

MOST PEOPLE ASSUMED I WOULD CONTINUE teaching once Anne and I had relocated to the house we bought in Seattle's Ballard neighborhood. They assumed I would find a way, despite my Parkinson's, to do adjunct teaching at one of the many colleges and universities in and around Seattle, or to teach a non-credit retirement enrichment seminar to local senior citizens, or to start my own book group at one of the branches of the Seattle Public Library, or to be a distance-learning teacher by teaching an online course in which I would never have to meet a "live" class, but instead teach remotely, via the interactive internet, to students scattered all over the country.

Nope. I had no desire to teach ever again. They say that once a king, always a king, but once a knight is enough. I've discovered that once a teacher, always a teacher, but forty years in the traditional classroom is enough. I had been there, done that for four decades at Lehigh University in Bethlehem, Pennsylvania, for a year as the Robert Foster Cherry professor at Baylor University in Waco, Texas, and for a year as a Fulbright professor at Sichuan University in Chengdu, China. If I wanted to keep teaching, why would I have retired in the first place?

Besides, with my Parkinson's diagnosis, how could I hope to succeed as a teacher, even if I had wanted to? I had gotten through those last two semesters at Lehigh without any of my students apparently knowing about my disease, but surely as my disease progressed it would more obviously impair my teaching.

Take voice. It is common for people with Parkinson's to grow weaker and weaker of voice until we can scarcely be heard at all. It is partly that our voice muscles atrophy, partly that the signals our brain sends to our lips and tongue get sidetracked before they get there so we lose our ability to articulate and enunciate. When I think about it, I can say the words "ar-tic-u-late" and "e-nun-ci-ate," but in practice they often come out more like "art-il-il-ate" and "nun-sate." I've always stuttered some, but my s-s-stuttering has gotten w-w-worse as my d-d-disease has p-p-p-progressed.

I have found that many people are embarrassed by my Parkinson's. They seem to assume that I am embarrassed by it and that I don't want them to notice it or mention it. In a sense that is true, of course. It is embarrassing to shake, to drop my fork, to stutter, to stumble, to drool, to walk more slowly than others, to "freeze" at doors, to fall down in public when I try to turn left or right. But I find that I don't at all mind talking about my disease if I sense that someone really wants to learn about it.

While I had no desire to teach another course on the *Canterbury Tales* or on contemporary Native American fiction, I found myself eager to share with others what I was learning about Parkinson's. In effect, I became a teacher again. As my disease matured, so did I. As my disease increasingly moved to the front-and-center of my life, I became less sensitive about what I assumed others were assuming about me as an old man with a scary disease. I grew less ashamed. I did not try to hide it. On the contrary, I became almost eager to reveal my association with it.

I never had to adapt my classroom teaching to the limiting disabilities of my disease. I was lucky enough to be diagnosed with Parkinson's near the end of my formal teaching career, so I had only a year of university teaching after I was diagnosed. I had to make no serious adjustments to my teaching style. I don't know that any of my students knew I had a brain disease. They may have thought I was kind of scatterbrained, or senile, or goofy, or just old. Perhaps they just thought all old guys shuffled when they walked and trembled when they handed back daily quizzes.

I am an incurable teacher with an incurable disease. I can't seem to shake either affliction. They are vastly different incurables, of course. Parkinson's is an oppressive medical condition anchored in genetics and chemicals and brain electricity. Teaching is an expressive psychological condition anchored in personality and insecurity and ego. To adjust to my retirement from good health I learned to read books, swallow pills, and exercise. Adjusting to retirement from teaching has been more a matter of teaching different subjects to different audiences.

One audience is myself. I have had to educate myself about Parkinson's. I have had to learn that Parkinson's happens when the brain stops making dopamine. I have had to learn that by the time the symptoms show up enough for a doctor to make a diagnosis, my dopamine levels are only twenty to thirty percent of normal, and they only get lower as time goes on. I have had to learn that, early on, people with Parkinson's lose their sense of smell and get constipated.

I have had to learn a whole new vocabulary—medical terms like "MAO inhibitors," "carbidopa/levodopa," "dopamine agonist," "idiopathic," "rasagiline," "substantia nigra," "subthalamic nucleus," "Co-Q-10," "DBS." I have had to learn new meanings of old terms like "freezing," "mask," "off-times," "designer disease," and "impulse control." As a teacher, I had become pretty good at finding and synthesizing new information, so I am a good pupil for myself.

Another audience is my doctor. I have learned that my

neurologist can help me only if I keep reasonably accurate records of my symptoms and my reactions to my various medications, and if I explain myself clearly—only if, that is, I teach her well. She knows Parkinson's from medical school and books and journals, but she has not had the disease. Each of us people with Parkinson's has his or her own unique blend of symptoms and reactions to medications. Because I'm the expert on my particular disease, I do best if I go to my appointments fully prepared with clear explanations of how I am doing and with well-formulated questions. I can educate her best if I prepare as carefully to teach her as I used to prepare to teach my classes.

For a recent (mid-June 2018) meeting with my neurologist, I went in with this list:

> **June 14, 2018**—Pete Beidler's troublesome symptoms:
> **Freezing FOG** (freezing of gait, stutter-stepping), especially
>> —in doorways
>> —when turning corners
>> —when carrying things
>> —in crowded rooms or restaurants
>> —on rough terrain or grass
>> —reaching out to prevent falls (sore shoulders)
>
> **Stumbling and falling**, especially
>> —at "off-times" (end of dose-period)
>> —after extended standing at my computer desk
>> —after sitting or lying down
>> —when talking while walking
>
> **Voice and speech** (stutter, soft voice, garbled words)
> **Drooling**, embarrassing, messy
> **Choking**, when I lie on my back (I mostly sleep on my side now)
> **Constipation**, frequent need for enema-assist, stool softener, and polyethylene glycol

Numbness in front part of feet, icy toes (neuropathy?)

Questions for neurologist:
1. Side effects of all the pills I take?
2. DBS (Deep Brain Stimulation)
         —any reason for me to reconsider it?
3. Does any medicine or surgery prevent freezing and
        falls?
4. At what point do we say, enough already?
5. How do people with Parkinson's die?
6. How does Washington State's Death with Dignity law
        work?

A third audience is the wider research community. I live in
Seattle, a city with a major university medical school, several
fine hospitals, an active VA hospital, and several Parkinson's
research centers. There is lots of research going on. Shortly
after I moved here I put my name on a "registry" of people with
Parkinson's who agree to be contacted when researchers need
volunteers. I have volunteered for studies involving speech
pathology, exercise, video gaming, genetics, and dementia. I
still don't like this disease, but I feel good knowing that my
having it may let me teach medical researchers about how to
treat it more effectively.

A fourth audience is the ordinary people who are as ignorant
as I was back in Pennsylvania. I don't go up to strangers and
say, "I'm a teacher. Let me teach you about Parkinson's!" But I
am happy to explain to people who show an interest in learning
something about my disease. All I really want from others is
their interest going in and their understanding going out. I do
not seek their help or even sympathy, but I do want them to
understand why it is important to me to manage on my own for
as long as I can. I want them to understand that I stumble funny
and mumble funny not because I am drunk but because I have
Parkinson's.

A fifth audience is my fellow sufferers with Parkinson's. When I first came to Seattle I signed up, with Anne's encouragement, for a Yoga for People with Parkinson's class at a nearby hospital. It was a pretty morose group. My ten yoga classmates had all been coming to the class once a week for a year, but they all acted like strangers, waiting glumly for the yoga master to arrive and start teaching. I decided to get to class early. As my classmates came in, I learned their names, and greeted them with a cheery, "Hi, Bill" or "How's Ron this week, Mary?" or "Did you get that truck fixed, Rich?" I was not their teacher, but I found myself doing what came naturally. Soon others started to come in early too, just because we had fun chatting. I brought in a deck of cards and several of us early-arrivals started playing a dumb card game called Peanuts. Then I brought a bouncing ball in to toss around as warm-up before the yoga master showed up.

One day I asked one of my classmates, a Hungarian woman named Maria, if she was a good cook.

"The best," she replied.

"Did you ever think of inviting the class to come over to your place for lunch after yoga class?"

"When do you want to come?" she replied.

Eight of us went. It was a lovely lunch.

Gradually we in the yoga class became our own Parkinson's support group, with garden parties, visits to shut-ins, welcomes to newcomers, an email list and a volunteer yoga-class secretary to keep the list up to date. We sent out messages, reminders, announcements, and so on. Gradually we added classes and now Yoga for People with Parkinson's has four classes a week at Northwest Hospital, with members who come once, twice, or even three times per week.

I am emphatically not the teacher of any of those classes, but perhaps I have helped a few of my classmates to become better students of yoga. I have not cured a single one of my classmates of Parkinson's, but perhaps I have helped a few of them to see that, far from being merely a disease that robs us of our abilities and our friends, it is a disease that can give us new abilities and bring us new friends.

4. You Have Parkinson's

"YOU HAVE PARKINSON'S."
      That is not what you wanted to hear. It is not what I wanted to hear when I got my diagnosis. I had seen what the disease did to my older sister: the slowness, the wooden gait, the tremors, the nausea after she took her meds, the freezing, the fumbling, the mumbling, the stumbling, the tumbling, the humbling. I wanted no part of it. You want no part of it, either.

But I have come to feel grateful for much of what my disease brings me. You may also.

I know, I know. Parkinson's has no friends. It is a disease no one wants. I didn't want it either, and I wish I didn't have it. I fully realize that you don't want to hear how fortunate you are to have this progressive, debilitating, degenerative, incurable disease. Right now the only bright side you can think of is that, well, you could have something even worse. You could have been diagnosed with liver cancer or with early-onset Alzheimer's. You could have had a paralyzing stroke or leprosy of the spinal column. You could have had an inoperable brain tumor or ruptured bilateral colostomic gangrene of the groin. You could have had Lou Gehrig's disease or a broken neck like the one that put Christopher Reeve into a wheelchair. You don't have any of those, right? Lucky you! But then you realize that having Parkinson's does not give you immunity from any of those could-have-been-worse medical conditions. You can still get those also. *Sigh.*

But wait. Let's put this diagnosis into perspective. There are approximately seven billion people alive in the world today. In a hundred years, all but a miserable few of those seven billion people will be dead, and those who are still alive will be fast approaching the grave. To be human is to be mortal. Before we wallow too deeply in the mire of self-pity brought on by our diagnosis, we should pause to remember that all seven billion of us, not just the ones with Parkinson's, are going to die. Most of us are going to die of or with something nasty. Naturally, we all want to live healthy and productive lives to a reasonably ripe old age—not *too* ripe or *too* old, of course—and we want to die suddenly, peacefully, and painlessly in our sleep with a smile on our lips. No muss, no fuss, no protracted care, no burdening of our families, no bankrupting medical expenses, no nursing homes, no hospice, no diapers, no grimaces, no regrets, no messes, no self-pitying.

But come on now. How many people do we know who have been so lucky? What makes us think we are entitled to be one of the very lucky, very few, who escape the agonies of a pre-death sickness and the indignities of a prolonged, messy, and expensive dying?

If we accept the reality that most of us are going to end our days with something awful, then Parkinson's is not such an unfortunate fate. The rest of this chapter is about the good things our diagnosis brings with it, the things we can be grateful for. No one likes this disease, but some of us can learn to love some of what it brings us. It is educational, slow-moving, relatively painless, actionable, treatable, sociable, shareable, and ennobling.

Educational. Parkinson's gives those of us who have it an amazing education. It teaches us all sorts of things worth knowing. By showing us how little control we have over our health, it teaches us humility. By showing how much control we do have over our Parkinson's, it teaches us optimism. By showing us that bad things sometimes happen to good people who have done nothing to deserve bad things, it teaches us forbearance. By showing us how much we can do in spite of the disease, it teaches us self-reliance. By showing us the difference between the things we cannot change and the things we can, it teaches us both wisdom and serenity. By showing that we must work harder and smile more when things get tougher, it teaches us grace. By showing us that we need to look past the gray shades to the splashes of color, it teaches us gratitude.

We can all learn from Michael J. Fox, who in his 2002 memoir *Lucky Man* wrote that "these last ten years of coming to terms with my disease [have been] the best ten years of my life—not in spite of my illness, but because of it." He insisted that being forced to deal with his Parkinson's had "profoundly enriched" his life and made him a far better man. He *liked* the person Parkinson's made him: "If you were to rush into this room right now and announce that you had struck a deal [...] in which the ten years since my diagnosis could be magically taken away, traded for ten more years as the person I was before—I would, without a moment's hesitation, tell you to take a hike" (B4, p. 6).

Slow-moving. By the time most of us are diagnosed with Parkinson's, the disease has been with us for at least a decade. That fact is emblematic of its slow progress. Think of all you have done in the decade before your symptoms made you aware of your disease. You can get even more done in the decade ahead because now you can grit your teeth, set your jaw, and focus your efforts.

The slow progression of the disease gives us time to do the things we put off doing before we were diagnosed: travel, visit friends, confess, make amends, do good deeds, write our memoirs, fall in love, whatever. I've been diagnosed for more

than a decade, and at seventy-nine can still do much of what
I used to be able to do at fifty-nine and sixty-nine. I still get
around some of the time without a walker or a wheelchair.
Jeanne, one of my friends, was diagnosed more than two
decades ago, and so does she.

I still write emails, articles, and books, I still read a lot, do
wood-carving and simple carpentry projects. Three summers
ago I helped my daughter rebuild her decaying barn. Three
winters ago I built a basketball court in my backyard for my
grandson. Because my meds make me drowsy, I don't drive
anymore, but by a combination of Ubering, Lyfting, Access
(a county shuttle service for seniors), generous friends and
neighbors, an indulgent wife, and concerned children and
grandchildren, I can get to just about every place I need to go in
the lovely city of Seattle.

Furthermore, Parkinson's has given me plenty of time to, as
they say, put my affairs in order. I've weeded out lots of books
and files, updated my will, signed end-of-life directives and
DNR (Do Not Resuscitate) documents (more on these directives
and documents in Chapter 20 below, "The Way Ahead"). I have
had the time to devise strategies for making these next months
or years as pleasant and as productive as possible for myself and
the wonderful family that my disease inevitably affects.

Painless. Parkinson's is almost painless for most of us. For
me the only pain so far comes in the leg cramps I occasionally
get at night when I am sleeping. When the cramps wake me
up I can usually get the pain to go away in a few minutes by
stretching out the toe or heel. If that does not work, I get up
and walk around for a few minutes, sit and read for a half hour,
then go back to bed. If I sit too long in the same position, my
lower back starts to hurt. The solution for me is not to sit too
long in the same position. When I travel by car I make sure we
stop every couple of hours so I can take a little walk. When
I fly I insist on an aisle seat so I can cruise up and down past
the bobble-heads. I now have my home computer on a stand-

up desk, thus easily avoiding the discomfort that comes from sitting too long hunched over my computer. Now I hunch over my computer standing up (more on the pain of Parkinson's in Chapter 11 below, "What Parkinson's Feels Like").

Actionable. People with Parkinson's can work individually or in groups to keep the disease more or less at bay. We no longer have to sit back and wait while the disease robs us. On the contrary, virtually everyone who works with this disease now recognizes that the very worst thing we can do is sit back and wait. As my friend Terry puts it, we need to take the *park* out of Parkinson's. We need to unpark ourselves. We need to introduce into our lives as many action verbs as we can think of: bike, box, build, carve, chop, climb, clip, cook, create, cut, dance, dig, drag, grab, grip, grope, hammer, haul, hike, hug, jerk, jitterbug, jog, jostle, juggle, kick, kiss, laugh, lift, move, mow, paint, patch, pedal, peel, play, prune, pull, punch, punt, putt, rake, row, run, scramble, scratch, sew, shovel, snorkel, tile, and, of course, walk, and Zumba. The more we move the more we can move. For how many nasty diseases are we allowed, nay, supposed, to keep on doing the things we most love doing? For how many nasty diseases are we so much in control of our own continuing health?

Treatable. Parkinson's is treatable. Neurologists now have in their arsenal an amazing variety of medicines they can prescribe. Chief among these is something confusingly called carbidopa/levodopa (sometimes known as L-dopa or dopa-dopa or by a brand name Sinemet). Parkinson's disease happens when the brain gradually and mysteriously stops manufacturing dopamine. Carbidopa/levodopa synthetically replaces that dopamine. I now take carbidopa/levodopa pills eight times a day. I also take something called a dopamine agonist (sometimes known as ropinirole or by a brand name ReQuip). These little pills help us folks with Parkinson's move and keep our balance.

When these medicines begin to lose their effectiveness—

as they will—or begin to produce unpleasant side effects, neurologists can recommend still other meds, or even surgery. One surgical procedure is called deep brain stimulation or DBS (more on this procedure in Chapter 5 below, "Your Parkinson's Team"). Another is a product that squirts medicine though a tube directly into your small intestine. For those of us willing or eager to try non-traditional and natural medicines, there are many options in addition to our other meds. One of those, for example, is to take a snuffle-it-up nasal spray called glutathione.

There is no known cure for Parkinson's, but several organizations, such as the Michael J. Fox Foundation, continue to fund the kind of research that allows us to hope that a cure of some sort may be not far in the future (more on this in Chapter 13 below, "The Cure for Parkinson's").

Sociable. Parkinson's responds well to human interaction. We can go it alone, if we like, but it is much more fun to go it along—that is, along with others who have the disease and so know from personal experience what Parkinson's is like. People who do not have Parkinson's often pity those of us who do. People who have Parkinson's do not pity one another. Rather, we feel empathy with one another. Most of the people I know who have Parkinson's respond positively to the fellow-feeling of others. We rarely complain to one another about our illness. We rarely give one another advice. It is enough to know that someone out there understands—from the inside—what we are experiencing (more on this in Chapter 6 below, "Parkinson's Support Groups").

One of the main reasons I like my Parkinson's is that it has introduced me to some wonderful men and women. Without this disease I would never have met the other delightful people I know who have the disease, folks like Bill, Nola, Judy, Ed, Rich, Mary, Maureen, Terry, Karen, Nan, Ruth, Pat, Dick, Richard, Brian, Vic, Stephen, Jennifer, Christine, Griggs, Jeanne, Corbin, Maria, Marty, Patty, Angelique, Katie, Ralph, Jeannie, Karla, Neil, Jerry, Glenn, Sam, Vicki, Kevin, Lucy,

Terry, José, Toby, Marty, Carol, Jude, Chuck, Marvin, Erin, Tom, Bob, Phyllis, Linda, Trudy, and so on and so forth. Without my Parkinson's I would never have met the amazing medical, research, and support people who work with people like me. I would never have met people like Lauren, Keeley, Deborah, Julie, Lindsey, Sujata, Meleah, Amy, Patty, Melissa, Jordan, Carin, Karen, Kristie, Joyce, Susie, Rosalind, Jennifer, Elli, Heather, Debbie, Peggy, Sean, Carol, Terry, Larry, Jean, Tom, Laurie, Sam, Lisa, Maria, Steve, Serena, Yolanda, Suzanna, BetteJane, Sydney, Jodi, Donovan, Rebecca, Susie, Jenny, Jordan, Sarah, Peter, and Jeanne. Thank you, Parkinson's, for bringing these amazing people into my life.

Shareable. Early in this chapter I announced that Parkinson's is educational because it teaches those of us who have the disease many good lessons. My point in this section is that our Parkinson's gives those of us who have it a wonderful chance to be educators, to share our knowledge and experience with others.

I spent most of my working life as a teacher. One of the gifts of Parkinson's is that it gives me—gives all of us who have this disease—a chance to teach our families and our friends how destructive it can be for us to waste our time and energy feeling sorry for ourselves, railing against the undeserved unfairness of it all, complaining as one after another of our abilities is taken away. Parkinson's gives us a chance to teach our families and our friends how to greet adversity with dignity, with grace, with courage, and with a sense of humor.

We can teach by volunteering, as I do, in local university classes. I have, for example, given short talks in Dr. Kristie Spencer's graduate seminar on neurogenic motor speech disorders at the University of Washington. I go in and talk for ten minutes so that her students can see—that is, hear—what happens to the voices and speaking habits of people with Parkinson's. I have several times agreed to be examined by Patti Matsuda's graduate students in physical therapy at the

University of Washington. For most of these students I am their first "real" patient. They talk to me, ask me questions, observe my gait, notice my posture, and give me balance tests. Then they recommend, under the watchful eye of a faculty supervisor, a list of exercises that might help me. These students do help me, of course, but I also help them to learn about Parkinson's.

We people with Parkinson's are uniquely positioned to help educate researchers seeking more effective treatments and a cure. We can volunteer for one of the many research projects that are underway around the world. We can participate in research studies that test the efficacy of various kinds of exercise and various kinds of medicine. We can donate our brains to doctors doing medical research on Parkinson's.

My brain has helped me to teach while I am alive. I take pleasure in knowing that after I am dead that same brain, simply because I have Parkinson's, can help me continue to teach in the coming decades. I am proud to imagine that, both alive and dead, I can help to find a cure for this disease that no one really likes. No one, that is, except some of us who have learned to try to embrace rather than fight Parkinson's, to grow up to it rather than be diminished by it, to share rather than conceal what we have learned about it, to love parts of it rather than hate all of it, to laugh defiantly at it rather than cringe fearfully before it.

Ennobling. Most of the people I know with Parkinson's disease do not waste much time or energy in the pity-pot—perhaps I should call it the PD-pot. The questions about how and why and where we got this disease and what it means for our jobs and our dreams—those questions soon fall away. They are almost immediately replaced with nobler questions about what our Parkinson's will eventually mean for our families.

I am, for example, concerned about what my Parkinson's has in store for me, but I have been pleasantly surprised to discover that I am more concerned about what my Parkinson's will mean for my lovely wife Anne. I think I can handle what lies ahead for me. I am not sure I can handle what lies ahead for Anne. I know, I know, we both signed on "for better or for worse, in sickness and in health" more than a half-century ago. I like to think that in some small ways I have made Anne's life a little better. I do not like to think that I may soon be making her life a lot worse. I do not like thinking what that may mean for Anne in the months or years ahead as my Parkinson's makes me increasingly disabled (more on this in Chapter 20 below, "The Way Ahead").

Perhaps "ennobling" is too strong a term for the realization that I am less concerned about what Parkinson's will do to me than about what it will do to the people I care most about. Perhaps what I should be saying here is that Parkinson's gives us *and* our families the opportunity to be noble as we face *together* the uncertainties and opportunities that lie ahead.

Your Parkinson's will grow in you, but it will also grow on you. Most important, your Parkinson's will grow you.

Remember to say "Thank you" to your amazing family who help you in so many ways, to your amazing new friends who let you know in so many ways that you are not alone, to your amazing Parkinson's team, and to your amazing disease for giving you and your family a chance to behave nobly in the years ahead.

Thank you. All of you.

5. Your Parkinson's Team

So NOW YOU KNOW. YOU HAVE PARKINSON'S. That means that in the coming weeks, months, and years you will encounter many individuals and groups of people who will together make up your Parkinson's team. Most of them will not know each other. All that they have in common is you. It falls on your broad shoulders, then, to be the team captain. Here are some of the people on your team.

Your care partner is the person (often referred to as your "caregiver") who will be your main at-home helper and facilitator. I have been super-fortunate to have Anne, my wife of more than half a century, as my care partner. She comes with me to visit others on my team, orders my medicines, drives me places I need to be, schedules the Access vans that pick me up. Of course, I do things for her, too, because I am her care partner. I go with her when she has a macular degeneration checkup, I encourage her to call her doctor when she has what may be another urinary tract infection, deal with car mechanics, balance our checkbooks, do our income taxes. For others with Parkinson's, the care partner is a parent, or a child, or a sibling, or a neighbor, or a friend with or without this disease. For others it is a paid companion or someone at a county nursing home. I know many people with Parkinson's who succeed at managing their own affairs for a long time. I know others who, in addition to taking care of themselves, have also to take care of an ailing spouse or parent. We usually find a way to manage, somehow. For most of us our initial professional contact is with our family doctor, often called our primary care physician.

Your primary care physician is the generalist whom you will probably consult first to ask about your tremor or your shuffling gait or your slowness or your constipation or your inability to smell or whatever it was that first caused you to seek out a professional medical opinion. If you are lucky, your family doctor knows your medical history and treats your everyday illnesses. He knows you well and probably has treated you for some time for routine medical issues: colds, flu, migraines, joint pain, sprained ankles, nasal congestion, menstrual or urological issues, skin blotches, bee sting reactions, allergies, blood pressure issues, prostate and colon issues, whatever. If your primary care physician sees reason to suspect Parkinson's, he will usually refer you to a neurologist or perhaps to a particular kind of neurologist known as a movement disorder specialist.

Your neurologist or movement disorder specialist will ask you a lot of questions and observe you carefully. There is no chemical test for Parkinson's disease. That is, she cannot send a vial of your blood or your urine to a lab, read the results, and know right off that you have—or do not have—Parkinson's. She will have to rely instead on a careful physical examination and close observation of your movements. She will test your strength, your limb coordination, your flexibility, and your balance. She will ask you to tap your toes on the floor. She will ask you to tap your right index finger rapidly against your right thumb, then do the same for the left hand. She will watch you walk down the hall to see if you swing your arms and how you manage turns. After an hour with you, she will have a pretty good idea whether you demonstrate early-stage Parkinson's. If she thinks that you probably do, she may have you take a pill and walk around the block for a half hour, then come back in and redo some of the tests. If the pill helps, that is a pretty good indicator that you have Parkinson's. Even if she is pretty sure that you have Parkinson's, she may not prescribe medications yet. She will probably, as your disease progresses, prescribe low, then eventually higher, doses of medicines with funny names like carbidopa/levodopa and rasagiline and ropinirole. Meanwhile, she may recommend that you start a regular exercise program. She may refer you to a physical therapist.

Your physical therapist will watch the way you walk and turn corners. He may suggest that you take longer strides and swing your arms when you walk. He may urge you not to pivot when you turn a corner but to take wider steps. He may give you a series of exercises to do a certain number of times a day for a specified number of days and then come back again. He may suggest that you try a different kind of shoe, or pick your feet up when you walk, or try using a cane, a walker, or a rollator (a four-wheeled walker) with a built-in seat. If you "freeze" when you walk he may suggest that you try a laser device—that is, a cane or a walker that provides you with a red laser line on the floor in front of your feet to prompt you to consciously step up over it and so begin to move forward again. You may decide that you want to see if a naturopathic doctor can help you.

Your naturopathic doctor will ask you lots of questions about the food you eat and the vitamins and dietary supplements you take. She may clip a bit of your hair and send it, along with a vial of your blood, to a laboratory for analysis. Then she may call you back in and suggest that you take a series of vitamins and other supplements. She may suggest that you eat more fresh fruits and vegetables, that you avoid carbohydrates and dairy products. She will not tell you that she can "cure" your Parkinson's, but she may say that if you do what she urges you to do, you will feel better and will give yourself the best chance of slowing the disease progression. Eventually, she or your movement disorder specialist may suggest that you consider one of several surgical options. If you decide to explore that possibility, you will need to seek the advice of a neurosurgeon.

Your neurosurgeon will give you a careful examination, both on and off your regular meds, and see how you react to them. Depending on your age and general health and the symptoms you show both on and off the meds, he will then, after consultation with others, decide whether you are a promising "candidate" for surgery. The main surgery now being performed on Parkinson's patients is called deep brain stimulation (DBS). It involves drilling two round holes the size of dimes into your skull and placing tiny wires deep into your brain stem. A couple of weeks after that part of the surgery, he will hook the wires up to small battery packs that he has implanted into your chest. The batteries send electrical impulses through the wires to electrodes spaced out along the wires. Those electronic impulses then act as a kind of pacemaker for the brain. There are, obviously, certain risks with such surgery, but the procedure can sometimes do good work, particularly in controlling tremors.

These folks are the core of your Parkinson's team. Others on your team may be **social workers** who can help guide you through the confusing governmental and medical organizations in your area, **psychologists** who can help you deal with anxiety and depression, **contractors** who can install ramps and guard rails in your home, **occupational therapists** who can show you how to make your home safer or your computer more convenient, **speech pathologists** who can help you talk louder and more distinctly, **neuro-ophthalmologists** who can help if you see double images, **yoga masters and tai chi instructors**, who can share with you the benefits of certain movements, stretches, and poses, **reference librarians** who can help you locate books, **dance therapists** who can show you how music can help you move more safely and gracefully, **trainers** at one or more exercise gyms who can show you some exercises that will help you, **legal and financial advisers** who can help you plan for some of the non-medical ramifications of Parkinson's, **administrators** at one of several organizations like the APDA (American Parkinson's Disease Association), and the NWPF (Northwest Parkinson's Foundation), **research scientists** who may invite you to be a volunteer in some research project they are engaged in, **neighbors and friends** with (or without) Parkinson's, and the **fine men and women** you meet in Parkinson's support groups. Your Parkinson's team is a shifting set of people who care about you and want to help you. Most of them don't know anyone else on your team. They will expect you, with the help of your care partner, to coordinate the efforts of members of your team and the help they can offer you, individually and collectively. You are the leader, the head honcho.

Take charge, boss!

6. Parkinson's Support Groups

L IKE MOST OF US, I WAS devastated by the diagnosis that I had Parkinson's. I was angry, distraught, self-pitying, and lonely. What had I ever done to deserve such a miserable disease?

Now, more than ten years later, I have discovered that Parkinson's is not such a devastating disease after all. Or, more precisely, I have discovered that I do not need to be devastated by it. I have several strategies for coping with my Parkinson's. I try to get lots of exercise. Until recently, I have been able to walk several miles every day. I went to the local gym several times a week, walked the treadmills, attended exercise classes, rode stationary bikes, danced Zumba. I visited several physical therapists and tried to follow their directions: "pick your feet up," "take longer strides," "heels down first," "knees higher." I listened to my team of neurologists at Swedish Hospital, Cherry Hill. I took the meds they recommended. I also went to a naturopathic doctor and followed her suggestions—well, most of them. I took a lot of pills, knowing that they supplied some of the chemicals that Parkinson's kept my brain from producing.

Perhaps what has helped me as much as the pills and the exercise and the professional advice is the knowledge that I have the support not only of an amazing wife and family but also of the many support groups that are available in the Seattle area. Most of these groups meet once a month. A typical support group meeting focuses on a speaker who makes a presentation of some sort and then invites questions. Sometimes a meeting is just a "discussion meeting" where members of the group raise issues and concerns and invite others to comment.

My first support group was started in the town of Edmonds, fifteen miles north of Seattle, by Nola Beeler. She and the others who attended—some with walkers, some in wheelchairs, some with spouses or other care partners—made me feel immediately that I was not alone with this disease. Others knew from experience what I was feeling, what frightened me, what amused me. We all helped each other with suggestions, with information, with empathy and—let's admit it—with love.

Nola eventually moved away from Edmonds, but the support group she started was next facilitated by Carol and Emilio Aguayo. Under their leadership, the monthly meetings continued to attract around fifteen or twenty participants. Not all support groups persist. The one at Swedish Hospital Cherry Hill was brilliantly facilitated by Peggy Shortt, but dissolved after a few years. A larger support group meets once a month at Horizon House in downtown Seattle. Facilitated for years by social worker Carin Mack, it has since had several other leaders and attracts as many as thirty or forty participants. I have recently started attending a Parkinson's support group that meets under the guidance of a social worker named Suzanna Eller. I go whenever I can, and always come away feeling wiser, mellower, and less alone.

We all know, of course, that Parkinson's is a highly individualized disease. There are some symptoms more or less common to most people with Parkinson's—stiffness, slowness, tremors, uncertain balance, soft voices, constipation—but we all display somewhat different mixes of those and other symptoms, and we all move along with our disease at somewhat different paces. Support groups let us know that, whatever our symptoms and whatever the pace of progression, we are part of a community of individuals who understand what it is like to have this disease.

Any group that brings people with Parkinson's together can become a support group. My own best support group is not officially a Parkinson's support group at all. It is my Yoga for People with Parkinson's class. Originated a decade ago by Tim Seiwerath, it is now (winter, 2019) taught by Peter Lynch. I attend the class twice a week at Northwest Hospital. Some of my closest friends in Seattle I first met in that class. We greet each other, listen to each other, share information with each other, console each other, offer rides to each other, tell stupid jokes to each other.

No support group can cure Parkinson's, but any support group can offer information, comfort, understanding, and solace to those of us who wait, patiently, for the cure that we want to hope will someday help us or others who will be diagnosed in the months and years to come. It is good to know that we are not alone with our worsening symptoms. If it is unfortunate to have Parkinson's, then surely it is more than doubly unfortunate to have it in isolation. To know that we are not alone with our disease makes it, if not fun, at least *more* fun.

If you live in an area with no support groups, start one. You may think there are not enough people with Parkinson's in your area to make up a support group, but ask around. Talk to doctors, senior centers, hospitals. You'll be surprised.

7. Ten for David

[In the summer of 2016 I gave the opening remarks at a seminar on treatment options for Parkinson's disease at a Northwest Parkinson's Foundation "PD University." It was held at a retirement community in central Seattle. I later was invited to publish my remarks in the Parkinson's Post, *the newsletter of the Northwest Parkinson's Foundation.]*

ON MONDAY I LEAVE FOR KANSAS CITY to visit a relative named David. About a month ago David was diagnosed with Parkinson's disease. I assume that he has been surfing the web for information about his disease, as I did a decade ago when I got my diagnosis. If he did, he will have read all sorts of nasty things about Parkinson's:

"No cure," "progressive," "degenerative," "muscle deterioration," "stiffness," "loss of motor function," "loss of brain function," "loss of ability to speak clearly," "difficulty swallowing," "constipation," "tremors," "dopamine deficiency," "postural instability," "freezing of gait," "loss of balance," "falling," "urinary urgency," "clinical depression," "cognitive dissonance," "sexual dysfunction," "compulsive behavior," "sleep disorders," "nocturia," "dementia."

And so on. After reading such descriptions of what can lie ahead for him, David will probably not be in the mood to hear what I am trying to say, but here are ten things I hope to have a chance to tell David:

1. Sure it's bad, but it's not as bad as you might imagine. We are all destined to get something, and there are many worse diagnoses than Parkinson's. Parkinson's is not for most of us a painful disease and it moves slowly. For many years to come, David, you will be able to function pretty much as you always have.

2. Let the disease help you focus your energies. Since you know that troublesome times lie ahead, use that fact to help you decide how you want to use these good years. Get started on your bucket list. Travel. Write. Visit old friends and neglected family members. Make peace with old enemies. Clean out your attic, garage, closets, and files. Appoint someone as your durable power of attorney for financial matters. Fall in love.

3. Always take one more step. Let no step be your last. Plan activities that make you move—yoga, biking, hiking, dancing, boxing. Walk to where you want to go—to the bus stop or to the gym or to the restaurant. As you walk, listen to the birds singing, to the wind in the trees, to the happy laughter of little children on the playground. If you sit around and wait for your Parkinson's to get worse, it will get worse faster. Don't give it a chance to immobilize you.

4. Don't whine. When your sister asks you how you are, tell her you are "doing pretty well, thanks, can't complain." If she asks you a second time—"No, really, David, how *are* you?"— go ahead and tell her something like, "Well, I'm doing pretty well, all things considered. My biggest frustration is that it is almost impossible for me to type now. My left fingers just don't do what I tell them to." Tell her more, if she asks, but keep in mind that not many people want to hear about *all* your woes unless they think they can help. They usually can't, so be stingy with your complaints.

5. Find others with Parkinson's. Find or start a Parkinson's support group. No whining is necessary when you are surrounded by others with the disease. They will *know.* They will *understand.* My Parkinson's disease has introduced me to many wonderful people who *know* and *understand.*

6. Be a part of the cure. Chances are that not far from where you live a neurologist or medical researcher is looking for people like you who have Parkinson's. These researchers need volunteers to help them try new treatments or medicines. Help yourself and others. In Seattle we have a Parkinson's Registry that gives people with Parkinson's the opportunity to volunteer for all sorts of studies. Since my diagnosis, I have volunteered for research projects on voice therapy, video-gaming, physical therapy, genetic studies, and dementia studies. For one study I wore a Fitbit watch and electronic socks that recorded my activity levels. I was amazed to discover that in the two-week period I wore that stuff I had walked a total of eighty-five miles. You didn't ask for your Parkinson's, but now that you have it you can be a help to researchers who are studying the disease.

7. Think about how you want to die. Washington State is one of the few states that give you meaningful legal choices about how long you live and how you want to die. What about Kansas? Have a talk with your doctor and members of your family about end-of-life issues, under what circumstances you want be revived, how you feel about breathing machines and feeding tubes and palliative care. Sign an advance directive to let your doctors and your family know what you want the end of your life to be like. What about your remains—burial or cremation? Appoint someone as your legal durable power of attorney for health care decisions, authorizing that person to be your agent in decisions about your medical care.

8. Think about how you want to live. Set an example to

others. Be cheerful. Be more grateful for what you have than angry about what you've lost. This is your chance to be a hero, to show some true grit, to demonstrate grace under pressure.

9. Think about what you can do to make life as pleasant as possible for the people around you. You have it in your power to make life miserable for the people who, out of love or duty, want to help you in any way they can. Reward them for caring about you. Reward them for caring *for* you. Reward them for caring. Michael Kinsley said in a book that he published recently, in the twenty-fifth year since his Parkinson's diagnosis: "If you want to be remembered as a good person, then try to be a good person" (B3, p. 14).

10. Remember to laugh. As you know, the topic of this seminar is "Treatment Options for PD." As you probably know, there are several surgical options for people with Parkinson's. One of them is called deep brain simulation (DBS). That involves drilling two holes in your skull and inserting electrodes deep into your brain, then connecting those wires to batteries sewn into your chest. But that is just one surgical option. Let me tell you about the doctor who got Parkinson's, which as you now know is non-symmetrical. The disease affected mostly his left side, so he decided to treat his disease as if it were a kind of gangrene. To keep it from spreading to his other side he got his surgeon friends to surgically amputate his left arm and leg. It worked! I am happy to report that he is all right now.

So, David, follow my advice and you'll be all right.

8. What's So Funny?

WE DON'T HAVE TO BE PATCH ADAMS to know that laughter is good for us. The technical name for the science of laughter is psychoneuroimmunology. Psychoneuroimmunologists have proved that laughter can be effective in helping all sorts of patients recover from or deal with dire medical conditions. Researchers have shown that laughter can lower blood pressure, reduce stress, and stimulate the immune system. Laughter also releases our body's natural painkillers and gives us an overall sense of feeling better. Research shows that laughing fifteen minutes each day can prolong your life.

You may ask what people with Parkinson's can possibly find to laugh at. Actually, there is plenty for us to laugh at. After all, we walk funny, we talk funny, we eat funny, we drool funny, we fart funny, we get out of a chair funny, sometimes we fall funny, and when we have dyskinesia we flail funny. Dyskinesia is the technical term for the uncontrolled twisting and writhing and flailing of the limbs and torso that some people with Parkinson's exhibit. My advice is that you should never go to an auction if you have dyskinesia. You'll wind up buying everything on the docket.

I was really angry when my neurologist told me, "You have Parkinson's." "That can't be right," I told her. "I want a second opinion!" "All right," she said, "you're ugly, too."

Actually, Parkinson's is known to strike the most beautiful, the smartest, the most creative, and the kindest people in the world. If we don't find a cure soon, the world will soon be populated only by ugly, stupid, pedestrian, and cruel people.

Some folks find that acupuncture helps with their Parkinson's. I tried it, but for me it was not a jab well done.

Parkinson's slows me down. I used to be fast; now I'm half-fast. The only thing I do fast anymore is fall down the basement steps.

The other day I forgot to take my pill case with me. I stumbled into a Bartell's and said to the pharmacist, "I need some Sinemet." "Yes, sir," he said, "walk this way." He scurried off down the aisle to the pharmacy window. "If I could walk that way," I shouted, "I wouldn't need the damn Sinemet!"

I found out the other day that Parkinson's is a neurodegenerative disease caused by toxins in the environment. That's just a fancy way of saying we get it from toilet seats.

Parkinson's can be tough on a marriage. Tom has Parkinson's. He and his wife Janice went for marriage counseling. The counselor invited them to talk about what bothered them most about each other. "I'll go first," Tom said. "Two things really annoy me about Janice. One, she pushes me around all the time and two, she talks behind my back!" The counselor said, "Janice, would you like to respond to those charges?" "Yes," she said. "What the hell does Tom expect in that wheelchair?"

Do I believe in sex on the first date? Of course I do. At my age, and with my disease, there may not be a second.

People sometimes ask me what it is like to have Parkinson's. I tell them it is a lot like puberty: your voice changes, you feel awkward, you fumble around in the dark, your fingers quiver when you least want them to, and you have trouble with buttons.

I feel a special affinity for calendars, maybe because the days, like mine, are numbered.

Actually, I almost never think about dying. That's the last thing I want to do!

As a matter of fact, Parkinson's itself will not kill you. Instead, you choke to death on all the pills your doctors make you take.

I know I am supposed to get a lot of exercise, but I don't. It makes my beer spill.

We all know that people with Parkinson's need to get a lot of exercise. My neurologist urged me to enroll in an exercise class at a local gym. Realizing that I had gotten way out of shape, I signed up for an aerobics class at the nearby YMCA. The first day I bent, twisted, gyrated, jumped up and down, and perspired for an hour. By the time I got my leotards on, however, the class was over.

My neurologist told me that I am not a candidate for deep brain stimulation. "Why not?" I asked her. "Because your brain," she said, "is too shallow."

I went to my neurologist last week and said, "You gotta help me, Doc, my Parkinson's is making me shrink. Every day I am smaller than the day before. You gotta help me right away. I'm going to disappear if you don't do something right now." The doctor examined me. "Well, Doc," I said. "What did you find out? Tell me now. I gotta know right now what you can do to stop my shrinking!" The doctor replied, "Pete, you're going to have to learn to be a little patient."

At first I wondered why they call Parkinson's a "movement disorder." Then I got constipated and I knew: "Oh, that kind of movement!"

When I arrived in Seattle I got a job as a seismologist, but I was fired in a week because I kept announcing that we were having an earthquake.

My second job worked out better. I worked in a soda fountain making milkshakes.

Last week the Seattle Mariners—our professional baseball team—gave free tickets to people with Parkinson's. I went and was there when Kyle Seager hit that bases-loaded homer in the eighth. At first I couldn't figure out why the ball kept getting bigger and bigger—and then it hit me.

At that same game I went to one of the concessions stands and ordered five glasses of beer. I guzzled them down right away, one right after the other. "Wow!" the server said. "I never saw anyone drink five beers so fast! What's the rush?" I replied, "You'd drink that fast if you have what I have." He said, "What do you have?" "A dollar," I said.

Parkinson's usually causes insomnia. Last night I stayed up all night trying to figure out where the sun had gone. And then it dawned on me.

I want to tell a story. You see, the last couple of days I have been feeling really bad—feverish, dizzy, bed-bound, no appetite, couldn't sleep. I could scarcely make it to the toilet without losing consciousness. This morning as I lay there thinking that I must surely be dying, I smelled the most wonderful fragrance coming out of Anne's kitchen downstairs. My heart swelled up with love, because that smell meant that Anne was making my all-time favorite oatmeal-and-raisin cookies. I stumbled out of bed and made my way to the stairway and, holding onto the rail with both hands, I slowly hobbled my way down to the kitchen. When I got to the kitchen door I beheld, cooling on the counter, a couple of hundred of my most favorite cookies. "What a wonderful wife Anne is to make me all those delicious cookies," I said to myself as I stepped to the counter. I reached out to retrieve the nearest cookie, when all of a sudden a spatula slapped into the back of my hand. "Oh, no you don't," Anne said. "Those are for the funeral!"

Okay, that's your fifteen minutes of laughter for today. So you have Parkinson's. Learn to be a little patient. Learn to deal with it—gracefully, gratefully, and gleefully.

9. The Rain Is Shining

[The staff of the Northwest Parkinson's Foundation invited me to write a short essay about Parkinson's and Thanksgiving for the November 2016 NWPF Parkinson's Post. *This is what I came up with.]*

FOR PEOPLE WITH PARKINSON'S, CELEBRATING THANKSGIVING can, like an old turkey, be kind of tough. If we have a debilitating, progressive, incurable disease, what in the world do we have to be thankful for?

Being with friends and families is nice and all, but it also invites envy and embarrassment. We are surrounded by happy, healthy people who remind us by their very presence that we are not one of them. No wonder they look so happy on Thanksgiving Day. They have lots to be thankful for, like the fact that they don't have Parkinson's.

They step lively without fear of stumbling. They play ping-pong without stepping on their own toes. They don't drop food off their forks. They don't have to worry that they will spill grape jelly on their yellow shirt. They don't have to wonder if their face is mask-like. They don't speak "words" that sound like "worms" or "warts" or "wzklrms."

But hold on, pal. Would we really, even if we could, trade places with any of those "happy" people out there? They may not have our disease, but perhaps they suffer from something worse: a crumbling romance, a demanding addiction, impending financial ruin, abuse, cowardice, whatever. Let's not waste time in envy. Whatever disease we have, the other guy could have something a whole lot worse. Or she could be far less capable than we are of dealing with what ails her.

Let's also not waste time worrying about embarrassment. To be sure, everything we do on Thanksgiving has the potential to make us blush or cringe. Will we trip on that rug? Will we lurch forward when reaching out to hug someone we haven't seen for a year? When we open our mouths to shovel in a piece of mince pie, will a shiny sliver of drool come down to welcome it?

Remember, most of us are among friends on Thanksgiving. They will try hard not to be embarrassed by our embarrassment. They will try to include us in their awkward conversations, offer to bring us an appetizer that looks like oyster snot on a piece of toasted pig-ear. They will offer to help us remove our coat without calling attention to the fact that we need help removing our coat.

They are kind people. They will not let us get away with isolating ourselves. They will work hard to include us. We appreciate that they work so hard to include us, but we are embarrassed by their kindness. The last thing we want is to ruin their Thanksgiving by putting a damper on their good times. This is supposed to be a happy day, and we don't want to mess it up for them. We don't want to embarrass them with our clumsiness.

So what should we do? If we drop our dinner roll, we should roll with it. If our spoonful of cranberry sauce shakes when we lift it onto our plate, we should shake it off. If we spill gravy on our fly, we should swat that fly. If the gravy stain on our pants looks dark, we should make light of it: "Hey, at least it's not on the back!"

If we refuse to be embarrassed, no one else will be embarrassed either. If we spend a lot of time worrying about making fools of ourselves, we'll wind up spending a lot of time making fools of ourselves.

We need not be embarrassed by who we are or what disease we have. We need not wish we were someone else. We need to be thankful for the person we are and welcome the special guest, Mr. P., who has invited himself along to our Thanksgiving dinner.

On this special day, we need to remember all the things we have to be thankful for, like the new friends this disease has brought into our lives.

The sun is shining on this Thanksgiving Day. That sunshine is lovely here in the Northwest. Think of all those millions of people in the world's deserts for whom the shining sun is a blistering sun. It does not warm them, it scorches them. It does not grow their crops, it withers them.

Or maybe it is raining on this Thanksgiving Day. If it is, think of it as a shining rain that makes things green and replenishes those mountain reservoirs that supply us with drinking water all summer long. Think of all those millions of parched people who would die for that rain, or who may die without it. We should be thankful for the shining sun and the shining rain.

We can eat a locally grown organic Honeycrisp apple for breakfast. Most people in the world cannot.

We can have a newspaper delivered to our door—even on holidays. The front page reminds us to be thankful that we live in a nation where our vote counts—and so do the votes of people who disagree with us and vote idiots into office.

On this, the most American of American holidays, we have friends and relatives to spend the day with. Think of all those homeless, incarcerated, or enlisted Americans who don't, and who have no special food to eat and no special table to eat it at. Think of all those people all around the globe who have never heard of Thanksgiving and who would envy us if they had.

Thanksgiving gives us the opportunity to teach our friends and family, by our own example, how to deal with an unfortunate deal, how to smile through our mask, how to love what we have rather than wish we didn't have it.

Thanksgiving gives us the opportunity not to whine. Thanksgiving gives us the chance to take what life offers without, like Captain Ahab of the *Pequod*, demanding revenge against a white whale named Moby Dick and dragging the whole crew down with us as we seek that revenge.

Thanksgiving gives us a chance to show to others our courage and our gratitude for the good fortune we have been blessed with.

Thanksgiving gives us a chance for a day to stop fighting our disease and start embracing it.

A Thanksgiving holiday gives us a chance to remind ourselves that the word *holiday* comes from the words holy and day. Thanksgiving is a holy day. We can keep it holy by being thankful that we have such a good life, such a good family, such good friends, such good food, such good rain, such a shining disease.

10. My Parkinson's Friends

[Sung to the tune of "My Favorite Things" from the Rodgers and Hammerstein Broadway musical, The Sound of Music.*]*

Walking up stairways I frequently stumble,
Walking down sidewalks I take a bad tumble.
Walking bent over with too-tight hamstrings—
    These surely are not my favorite things.

Eating at diners I spill my clam chowder,
When I try talking my friends say, "Talk louder!"
I'm driving an old car that I've filled with dings—
    These surely are not my favorite things.

Typing long emails with letters all jumbled,
I shout, "Anne, I love you," but she says I've mumbled.
I lose playing poker (my Queens yield to Kings)—
    These surely are not my favorite things.

    When I stumble,
    When I mumble,
    When I tumble bad,

I simply remember my Parkinson's friends,
And then I don't feel so sad.

Sitting all lonely in deep concentration,
Wondering what brought on this tight constipation,
Wishing these dry guts would flow like the springs—
    These surely are not my favorite things.

Turning the fan on rank air to expel it,
Thinking, "Why bother, I can't even smell it?"
I lose table tennis (my pongs come out pings)—
    These surely are not my favorite things.

Hand-writing long poems that no one can make out,
Trying to warm my stiff arm with a shake-out,
I walk like a zombie whose arm never swings—
    These surely are not my favorite things.

    My thoughts jumble,
    And I grumble,
    Am I going mad?
    But then I remember my Parkinson's friends,
    And they make me feel so glad.

11. What Parkinson's Feels Like

WE TEND TO ASSOCIATE ILLNESS WITH physical pain. Cancer hurts. Migraine headaches hurt. A broken hip hurts. Cracked ribs hurt. Burns hurt. A herniated disk hurts. It seems that when most people ask me what it is like to have Parkinson's disease, they really want to know where, how much, and how often it hurts. The answers to those questions vary with each person who has the disease, but for me the answers have mostly been nowhere, not much, and almost never.

Physical pain. For me, Parkinson's has never been particularly painful physically. I sometimes get leg cramps in the early mornings before I get out of bed or when I try a particularly challenging stretch in my Yoga for People with Parkinson's class. I can usually make that pain go away by stretching out the heel of the cramped leg. If the cramp persists, I get out of bed or out of my yoga pose and walk around a little. Usually in less than a minute the cramp is gone and I can crawl back into bed or move on to the next pose. One of my doctors suggested that I eat bananas and yellow mustard—not necessarily together—to help prevent the cramps. No big deal.

At times there is pain associated with the exercises I do to try to keep fit. Sometimes my shoulders are sore after I do too many pushups. Almost always my crotch is sore after an hour of vigorous pedaling on a stationary bike at the gym. Sometimes after a strenuous Rock Steady Boxing workout my arms and shoulders are sore.

In recent months (I write this in June of 2018), I have experienced some pain associated with my falls. I now fall several times a day. These are rarely dangerous full-out sprawl-falls, but I usually bang at least one knee when I fall. I usually try to prevent a full-out sprawl-fall by reaching out with one or both hands. As a result, my knees, shoulders, wrists, and fingers are often sore these days, but soreness is not really pain. In sum, I have no right to complain about the physical pain associated with my Parkinson's disease.

I am aware, of course, that some Parkinson's patients do suffer pain on a regular basis. Nick Pernisco puts it this way in his recent (2019) book: "Pain is something that we deal with when we have Parkinson's. I've definitely experienced pain from poor posture and bad walking form. I have dealt with lower back pain, hip pain, and muscle aches" (p. 131).

I am also aware that just around the bend there lurks for me the possibility of a *big* sprawl-fall that can result in a lot of physical pain, but so far I have been undeservedly lucky. More troublesome for me than physical pain is emotional pain.

Emotional or futurized pain. The important pain I have felt as a result of my Parkinson's disease is what I might call emotional pain. It is the pain of knowing that a really *big* sprawl-fall is surely going to come. It is the pain of what I call "futurizing"—that is, of projecting what my life will be like down the road as I grow increasingly helpless. Futurizing is imagining my life in a later stage of my Parkinson's disease. Futurizing is imagining how awful it will be when I am immobilized and confined to a wheelchair or bedridden and unable to dress, feed, or bathe myself. I imagine myself as a quivering, drooling, bedsore-scarred invalid who is a pain in the neck to his wife and his children. That is what my futurizing "future-eyes" see when they look ahead. It is not a pretty picture.

It is emotionally painful to imagine that the money Anne and I had hoped to bequeath to our children may instead get sucked away to pay the exorbitant costs of medical care for the helpless and useless old invalid I have imagined myself inevitably becoming.

But wait. Is it really fair of me to futurize? In the first years of my diagnosis, I experienced the emotional pain of realizing that the carefree and productive retirement years I had so looked forward to were not going to happen. I would not be able to write any more books, travel to any more exotic places, renovate any more old houses, or help our kids renovate their homes.

Well, a decade and more have slipped on by and most of that futurizing is still in the future. I quiver and drool some, but I still dress myself, still step into and out of the shower by myself, still walk on two feet, and still have no bedsores on my butt. I use a walker when I go out but still have not yielded to a wheelchair—except at the airport. I am a pain in the neck to Anne and my children, but I guess I always have been, and they don't complain.

As for the money, the stock and real estate markets have been good to us, and Anne and I still have as big a nest egg as we had in 2006, when I retired. In these past dozen years, I wrote eight books. Anne and I traveled to exotic places—several times to some of them—such as Alaska, Arizona, Pennsylvania, California, Belize, China, Hawaii, Lopez Island in the North Pacific and Prince Edward Island in the North Atlantic. We bought the rundown bungalow next door to our house in Seattle, renovated it, and rented it out. And Anne and I have helped all four of our children improve their homes.

So, how am I doing now, in 2018? Well, the emotional pain is still way worse than the physical pain. I still "futurize." I see what has happened to my Parkinson's friends as they one by one have had to give up their mobility, curtail their activities, and stay home more and more. Every so often I hear that another Parkinson's friend is being cared for at least some of the time by a professional healthcare worker or is moving—or being moved—to a retirement or nursing home. It pains me to realize that I may be the next in line for such a move.

When I feel that kind of pain, I say to myself: "Stop it, Pete, you're futurizing again! The future you used to fear has not come to you, and the one you fear now may not come to you either. If and when it does, you will deal with it as best you can. You don't need to deal with it now. Enjoy the present. The future will take care of itself."

Well, now, if I do not feel much physical pain and if I talk myself out of feeling emotional pain, what does Parkinson's feel like? There is no way to give a simple answer to that question. It is different for each of us with the disease, and for each of us with the disease, the way it feels when we are first diagnosed is different from the way it feels later on. But it is a good question and deserves an honest answer. I will answer it by describing what my own Parkinson's feels like now, in June of 2018, a dozen years after my diagnosis. To start, I feel immobilized.

Immobilized. Parkinson's for me lives up to its name as a "movement disorder." Parkinson's makes me feel frustratingly slow. It limits the way I move. Take driving. Sensing several years back that I was no longer a safe driver, I reluctantly hung up my keys and gave my trusty old Chevy Suburban away. I had been driving for sixty years, and driving that Suburban—which I had bought new in 1984—for thirty years. I knew that if I did not get out from behind the wheel, I would eventually cause a serious accident. Giving up driving was the right decision, but it made me feel suddenly immobile. How in the world was I going to get around town?

I replaced driving with walking and bussing. A few years ago, I walked forty or fifty miles a week—to the gym, to yoga, to Home Depot, to Parkinson's support groups, to the library, to the post office, to one of a half-dozen bus stops within two miles of our house in Seattle. I can no longer walk that far. Hey pal, you try walking fifty—or even two—miles with a walker!

Now I probably do manage to walk a couple of miles a week—one of them on a treadmill at the gym. I am a huge fan of the Seattle Metro bus system but riding the buses has become more and more problematic. It was not just that I could not safely walk to the bus stops. It was also that I could not count on being able to get safely on or off the buses without tripping over my walker.

My immobility continues. Now when I want to go somewhere, I usually have to ask Anne or one of the kids or grandkids or Uber or Lyft to drive me there. A real boon for me has been the almost-free, big white Metro Access vans that are subsidized by King County. These magnificent vehicles will pick me up in front of my house and take me wherever I need to go in the city of Seattle: to my yoga class at Northwest Hospital, to the VA Hospital, to the YMCA up in Shoreline, to the Rock Steady Boxing gym over in Northgate.

My major moving problem now is FOG—no, not the gray mist that Seattle is famous for, but "freezing of gait." For seventy years, when I wanted to move in a certain direction, my brain told my feet to walk or run or skip or dance in that direction and my feet obeyed immediately. For the last couple of years, however, my feet seem disconnected from my brain. My brain says, "Feet, move Pete to that bus stop over there so he can get on the bus that will take him downtown to the central library." Instead of obeying such instructions, my feet say to my brain, "Nope. We don't take orders from you anymore unless we feel like it, and we don't feel like it just now. Tell Pete to take another pill and to concentrate on moving one foot and then the other, and we'll see if we can get him to the bus stop."

Sometimes it works and I get on the bus with my walker, but if I have to change my stride, or step off a curb, or step aside to avoid a dog or a fire hydrant, my feet may stop moving.

Sometimes when that happens my body continues to move forward and I fall.

My feet are particularly resistant to letting me walk through a doorway. Doorways into or out of elevators are especially challenging, because they shut without reference to whether I have yet struggled through the opening. The spring-loaded automatic door closers on public toilets are similarly problematic. But *any* doorways, even doorways with the doors propped open or doorways with the doors permanently removed, can bring me up short. There are no doors on escalators. I can usually get on the escalator easily enough, but I tend to freeze at the top when I try to step off. Perhaps that is because I know that my freezing makes me a dangerous roadblock to those behind me on the escalator. Knowing that I must get the hell out of their way makes me freeze even more.

What does it feel like to have late-stage Parkinson's? It feels as if my legs are numb and disconnected from my hips. It feels as if my feet might stick to the floor and cause me to fall without warning at almost any time. It feels, in short, precarious.

Precarious. I cannot any longer with any confidence carry a plate of fried eggs across the kitchen in my own home because I might stumble and drop them.

It feels precarious to take tiny "stutter-steps" because the front or ball of my foot hits the ground before my heel does, and I can dangerously stumble forward.

It feels precarious to stand at the start of a crosswalk on a busy street corner waiting for the WALK sign to light up, and then when it does light up, stand there frozen and unable to take that first step. It feels even more precarious to get halfway across that busy intersection and then freeze, knowing that when the light turns, the cars and trucks will start moving toward me. Will the drivers see me? Should I try to go forward? Should I turn back? Or should I stay in the middle and wait for the next WALK sign to light up? That makes it sound as if I have a choice. I don't.

It feels precarious when I cannot lift my left foot more than a half-inch above the floor, cannot take long steps, cannot make my heel hit the floor before my toes do.

It feels precarious to freeze thirty inches before I get to my bed or my dining room table and so lurch forward with my sore arms out to break my fall.

It feels precarious to lurch from walls to counters to chair backs to door jambs so that I won't fall down as I move around my own house, but then sometimes I fall down anyhow.

It feels precarious to lean instead of walk. When I freeze three feet before I get to the car and cannot take another step, I compensate by leaning toward the car. Sometimes my hands and arms halt the lean, but sometimes I wind up down on my knees and then hold onto the car's door handle as I try to stand up. Either way it feels precarious.

I carry in my wallet a card that says:

> **I have Parkinson's disease. I am not intoxicated. If I stumble or fall, or if I talk with a slurred voice, it does not mean I am drunk. Please take me to a hospital or call my wife Anne Beidler at the number on the back of this card.**

To act like a drunk when I am perfectly sober is embarrassing.

Embarrassing. I feel embarrassed to tell a person I am walking with that I cannot talk and walk at the same time because if I don't think about each step, I will stumble and fall.

It is embarrassing that I cannot put the trash out or help Anne carry groceries in from the car.

It is embarrassing that I have to keep moving, because if I sit down for more than an hour I get so stiff that I can scarcely move. I feel a little like a shark that knows it will drown if it stops moving. But sometimes I just can't move.

It is embarrassing to see how much of my bowl of chili I dribble on the tablecloth.

It is embarrassing to enter a crowded restaurant and not be able to walk among the tables without leaning on the backs of other people's chairs. To be unable to walk out of a restaurant without making other diners stand up to let me and my walker get by is frustrating.

Frustrating. It is frustrating to realize that when I try to talk, especially on the telephone, people can't understand me.

It is frustrating to try to keep track of the thirty-odd pills I have to take every day.

It is frustrating to give up multitasking. I used to reach out and flip the light switch without thinking when I walked into or out of a room. Now I have to do it with conscious thought: "If I want that light turned on, I had better stop here and reach over and flip the switch, and then pick up my left foot and start walking again. Or maybe I should lead off with the right foot this time. If I try to flip the switch while walking, I'll probably find myself in a heap on the floor."

It is frustrating that, when I bring the *Seattle Times* in from the front porch in the morning, I have to throw it across to the dining room table where I will sit down to read it. If I try to carry it across the kitchen, I may fall down, and I have to keep my hands free to break my fall.

It is frustrating not to be able to carry things. My worst falls have been when I am carrying—a plate of spaghetti, a hammer, a knife, a glass of water, my cell phone. When I fall while carrying something, I try to keep the thing I am carrying from crashing to the floor. It crashes to the floor anyhow, but I am so intent on protecting it, or protecting the floor, that I forget to protect myself and wind up with another scabby knee, sore wrist, or throbbing shoulder. As my frustration grows, so does my sense of being isolated.

Isolated. Parkinson's makes me feel isolated. I have always enjoyed talking with people. For forty years, I made a living by talking—by teaching, by participating in conferences with students or colleagues, by working on committees, by presenting the results of my research at professional meetings. As my Parkinson's has progressed, however, it has taken my voice away. People can no longer hear me because my voice has lost its volume. People cannot understand me because my words run together. I mumble. I stutter. As a result, I have virtually stopped talking, stopped telling silly jokes—well, not entirely—stopped chatting with old friends and new acquaintances in coffee shops.

My sfigtin hzx gzken hig sld. *Oops*. What I meant to say is that my writing has taken a hit also. My left hand usually misses the signal that my brain sends, so my right hand has to hit the backspace key over and over. And over. What used to be a ten-minute email message now takes an hour to write—most of the hour being spent correcting the goofy-looking words and punctuation.

What, then, does late-stage Parkinson's feel like? I can speak only for myself, but it makes me feel immobilized, precarious, embarrassed, frustrated, and isolated. I sound like I am complaining, but I really do not mean to. These are mostly minor inconveniences. I feel immobilized, but I still get around. I feel precarious, but have had—as of this writing—no really bad falls. I feel embarrassed, but I have grown used to embarrassment and find ways to avoid the most embarrassing situations or to convert them into amusement. I feel frustrated, but not cripplingly so. I feel isolated, but have many indulgent friends who patiently speak with me and for me. I know many men and women who have far worse inconveniences to deal with. But I also know that things for me have grown steadily worse in the past several years and will continue to get worse in the months and years ahead. Years? Did I really say *years*?

I wrote earlier of talking myself out of worrying about the future: "Stop it, Pete, you're futurizing again! The future you used to fear has not come to you, and the one you fear now may not come to you either. If it does, you will deal with it as best you can when you need to. You don't need to now. Enjoy the present. The future will take care of itself." That kind of self-lecturing helps some, but sometimes my other self talks back: "Yes, Pete, but it is irresponsible to pretend that if you don't think about the nastiness that lurks up ahead for virtually all Parkinson's patients, you will leave a mess for others to deal with when that nastiness does come. Is that fair to them?" That kind of self-dialogue has led me to write Chapters 17, "Depression and Self-Deliverance," 18, "Starvation and Dehydration," 19, "The ABCs of Self-Deliverance," and 20, "The Way Ahead."

12. How You Can Help

PEOPLE WHO HAVE PARKINSON'S KNOW HOW fortunate we are if we have a family member—usually a spouse or a son or daughter—who helps us. Often called "care partners" or "caregivers," these stalwart individuals do all sorts of things for us: order our meds, provide us with meals, take us to doctors' appointments, try to cheer us up, take us to movies, make phone calls for us, do our laundry, clean up our spills, worry about us. They often do all these things and more for little reward except, as the disease progresses, the reward of more work and then still more. Care partners are often themselves made sick by the unremitting decline of the person it is their lot to care for. This chapter, however, is not addressed to our care partners, who know only too well how they can help us. It is addressed to other people—relatives, friends, and strangers—who kindly offer us their help.

"How can I help you?" Everyone with Parkinson's gets used to hearing variations of that question: "Are you all right?" "Do you need something?" "Can I call someone for you?" "Would you like me to cut that steak up for you?" "Maybe you've had enough to drink. Can I call you a taxi?" "Would you like me to shuffle those cards for you?" "Can I hold that jacket for you?"

"Have you thought about selling your home and moving into an assisted-living place with a good infirmary?" "Can you get up out of that low-slung chair by yourself, or can I give you a pull?" At first we hear these offers of help from family and close friends. As our disease progresses, however, we hear them from strangers. People with Parkinson's often do need help, but often we do not. This chapter is designed to offer some helpful advice to the many good people who want to help us.

If you want to help us, you need to understand that while people who have Parkinson's appreciate your offers of assistance, most of us would rather continue to do most things for ourselves, if only to prove to ourselves that we still can do most things for ourselves. Every time we have to accept help with something we used to do without help, we feel that we are a step closer to the total disability we know is coming. We love you for offering to help, and we accept as gracefully and as gratefully as we can when we do need your help, but the more we accept your help, the more obvious it is that we are slowly approaching the really bad time that lies ahead. If we say, "No, thanks. I need to do this one myself," please do not be hurt. We absolutely do mean the thanks, but sometimes we also absolutely do need to do this one ourselves. We know that you could do it quicker, and that we could do it better or more safely if we accept your help, but sometimes slower may be better if it lets us live independently for a little longer.

So, what can you do to help? Well, you can begin by asking me questions.

Ask me about my Parkinson's. It helps me to know that you are interested in my disease. I am happy to tell people some of what I have learned through my personal experience and my reading, but I am reluctant to walk up to people and proclaim, "I am Pete. I have Parkinson's. Let me tell you about my disease!" I *do* like it if you show an interest. Don't assume that it is a sensitive subject or a taboo topic. Some medical topics *are* taboo—"Where'd you pick up that case of gonorrhea?"—but

Parkinson's is not one of them for most of us who have it.

Ask me whether I need your help. There is a world of difference between, "Here, let me help you with that jacket" and, "Do you need help with that jacket?" You can generally assume that I know when I need help and what kind of help I need. Sometimes I just need a little time. Try not to be impatient with your patient. Try not to assume that because I have Parkinson's I must therefore need your help. Your interest helps me, but it is important for me to continue, as long as I can, to do for myself what I can do for myself. I know you are eager to help me, but sometimes I need you to stand down and just let me do it. Trust me to know my own limitations. If I want you to cut my steak or shuffle the deck for me, I'll ask you to. Really, I will. Well, most of the time really I will. In general, then, let me decide what I can do. Don't assume that because I have trouble walking I also have trouble climbing stairs or pedaling a stationary bicycle. I freeze a lot when I walk. I almost never freeze when I go up or down stairs or pedal a stationary bicycle.

Ask me how you can help Anne. Parkinson's is often more difficult for the care partners of people with Parkinson's than it is for the people with Parkinson's themselves. I try to do what I can for Anne, but you can help me by finding a way to be nice to her. Take her to lunch. Invite her to take a walk around Green Lake with you. Bring her a flower. Ask her how my disease— really, *our* disease—affects *her* life. Find a way to show her that you care about her. Tell her to take a day off and that you'll come and bring me a sandwich for lunch. I do what I can to make life easier and less exhausting for her, but it would be lovely for us both if you paid her some attention.

Ask *me* to help *you* with something. Most people with Parkinson's are either retired or are officially disabled. We have time and we have certain skills, but we feel increasingly useless. We know a lot and we can do a lot. I am, for example, a pretty fair carpenter and teacher and writer and game-player. It makes me feel good if I can help others. Instead of being asked only what I need help with, it's nice to be asked for my help or advice.

Be especially careful about helping me with walking, freezing, falling, and getting up. Don't pull me or my walker. If you see me struggling with FOG (freezing of gait), you naturally want to help me move when I can't make my feet go. It is best not to take my hand or arm or walker and pull me forward. If you do that, you will pull me right down. I need to use one of my tricks to try to get my feet moving again—count, step in place, use a metronome, whatever.

Don't try to hold my hand if we are walking. Wait until we get to a park bench to do that. When I am walking, I really need to keep my hands free to grab a nearby tree or break my fall if I trip. I love holding hands, but for me it is a pleasure fraught with danger.

Don't try to get me to talk when I am walking. When I am walking, I need to focus my full attention on the walking—picking up my feet, swinging my arms, putting my heels down first, taking long strides, watching for roots, raised pavers, potholes, water puddles, and anticipating in which direction that corpulent man up ahead—the one with the leashed Doberman—is going to go.

Sometimes, just let me fall, especially if I am falling forward. I've had a lot of experience falling forward, with so far nothing worse than banged up knees and sore fingers, wrists, elbows, and shoulders to show for it. If you grab my hand or arm to keep me from falling, you may be keeping me from cushioning my fall with that hand or arm. Or I may drag you down with me, causing you to get hurt. I don't want that. You don't need that.

Think of standing or walking behind me rather than in front of me. When I fall forward, I use my hands and arms to break my fall. When I fall backwards, I have no way to reach back to break my fall and I am more likely to smash my head on a curb or a pavement. If you are behind me when I *start* stumbling back, try to steady me by pushing me gently forward or, if I am already careening back, get out of my way or grab me under my armpits to break my fall. But look out for yourself.

Be a human handrail. If you sense that I am about to freeze or fall, offer me a steady, horizontal forearm. Be a portable human handrail. I may not take it, but it's nice to have the option.

If I fall, let me try to get up by myself. Remember that I've had a lot of experience falling down and getting up by myself. Don't just assume that I need help and grab the nearest arm and pull on it. I may need to have that arm free as I rebalance myself. Ask me if I need help. I'll tell you if I do. It may well be that what I really need is your stiff horizontal forearm at the ready to hold onto as I rise up.

Encourage me, compliment me, but please don't tell me what a great job I am doing in fighting my Parkinson's disease. I have read Nick Pernisco's recent (2019) *Parkinson's Warrior*. Pernisco makes a vigorous case for treating our disease as an enemy that is out to destroy us. He tells us to "fight like you are battling a fierce enemy—because you are! […] It's important to have a strategy for how to fight each battle" (p. xvi). Pernisco thinks Parkinson's is best thought of as an evil enemy consciously trying to destroy you: "The disease believes it can take over your life by taking over your body. […] Today we know how to fight back, and just like fighting back against any arrogant bully, it's well worth the challenge to put it in its place" (p. 24). Our only hope is to fight it at every turn: "Fighting back against the disease is what we do. We are Parkinson's Warriors!" (p. 34). I am not at all sure I agree with this kind of thinking. I have trouble envisioning a disease as an evil bully intent on destroying good people like me. Parkinson's is just a disease. I would rather you praised me for trying to get along with a difficult neighbor than for trying to annihilate a fiendish bully.

There are lots of little things you can do to help me.

Answer the doorbell for me if you are inside. If you are outside ringing the bell, give me an extra minute to get there. Some things just take me longer, like getting to the door when the doorbell rings.

In a restaurant, ask for a table near the door. I panic in tight spaces with lots of narrow turns. If I have my walker, it is almost impossible to maneuver between the tables. Other patrons are happy to stand up and stand aside to give me room, but I hate inconveniencing other people or holding them up. Pressure makes the freezing worse.

Hold the door open for me, especially doors with spring-loaded automatic door-closers, like the ones found on most public restrooms. Elevator doors are particularly troublesome to me because they are gateways to tiny and often crowded spaces that I have to turn to get into or that I have to turn around in to get out of. I almost always freeze as I approach an elevator door, so it helps me a lot if someone holds the door long enough to let me enter. But try not to stand in the doorway as you do so, since that narrows the opening even more. And as for revolving doors, you can be a wonderful help by finding an alternative entrance. If you've ever experienced FOG (freezing of gait) in one of those revolving things, you'd never want to enter one again either.

Don't follow me too close onto an escalator, because I may freeze at the top or bottom when I try to step off the moving stairway. I will need extra time getting out of the way of the stampede coming up or down after me. Let ten steps go by empty before you step onto the escalator to follow me. Try to keep others from getting on any of those steps right behind me.

Carry things for me. I need to keep my hands free to hold onto my walker or my cane or a handrail, or to lean against a wall or, if I stumble, to break my fall. I have taken to carrying a shoulder-strap satchel to hold the stuff I used to carry in my hands: my water bottle, my cell phone, my meds-case, a magazine or book, an apple. If you see me trying to carry something, especially something spillable or breakable—a bowl of soup, a stack of dirty dishes, a newborn grandson—by all means offer to relieve me of my burden.

Answer the phone for me. My voice has grown soft and stuttery. Almost no one can understand what I say on the phone, so I rarely answer the ring. If you hear the phone ring, it would be kind of you to answer it for me because I won't.

Text me. If you want to tell me something, please do not phone me. Instead, text me or email me.

Keep your sense of humor. Tell me some jokes. Laugh at my jokes. It is hard for me to stay cheerful when the people around me are looking all glum and serious and embarrassed and uncomfortable. People with Parkinson's tend to keep their sense of humor. Help us help others to see what is funny.

Play games with me. I like to play games, especially ones that move quickly (like peanuts or gin rummy) and don't require deep concentration (like chess or bridge). I love to play Scrabble, but I advise you not to play me because I always win. *Ha!* Work on a picture puzzle with me. Watch a movie with me. Watch the Mariners lose with me. Offer to shoot a couple of games of pool with me.

Offer me a ride. I used to drive, bus, and walk every place I needed to go: to the gym, to yoga classes, to the library, to the University of Washington, to the doctor. But then Parkinson's reality set in. My reaction time and my alertness when driving my Suburban grew problematic, and I decided to hang my keys up before I did someone or something damage. Then I took busses, but soon I had trouble getting on and off. Then I began freezing when I crossed streets. Getting places is now a major problem. Anne generously drives me. I take Access vans. I summon Uber and Lyft. But I always appreciate a ride and rarely turn one down.

Finally, do your best to understand why it does not help me to have you tell me that surely a cure for Parkinson's is right around the corner, and that all I have to do is keep the faith a little longer and wait for it (more on this in Chapter 13 below, "The Cure for Parkinson's").

13. The Cure for Parkinson's

THE HOPE FOR A CURE FOR Parkinson's disease has been around for a long time. More than two centuries ago, in 1817, a British doctor published "An Essay on the Shaking Palsy." Based on his observations of a half-dozen individuals, Dr. James Parkinson described the disease with what turned out to be remarkable accuracy. It starts, he said, with a tremor, usually in the hand or arm, then proceeds to bent-forward posture, difficulty walking, frequent falling, difficulty feeding oneself, problems chewing and swallowing food, drooling, constipation, difficulty speaking, and extreme tiredness. The malady, he said, is "of long duration" and "the unhappy sufferer had no prospect of escape"—that is, had no hope of being cured. The accumulated symptoms led to what Dr. Parkinson called "the wished-for release"—that is, the desire for death. By describing the disease and its various stages, he said, he hoped that future research into the malady "might be productive of relief, and perhaps even of cure, if employed before the disease had been too long established."

If he were alive today, Dr. Parkinson would probably be surprised to discover that the disease he called the shaking palsy had been renamed in his honor, but he would be more interested in finding out whether two hundred years of research into "his" disease had been "productive of relief" and "even of cure." He would no doubt be thrilled that medical researchers had been able to offer sufferers some temporary relief from some of the symptoms of the disease that carries his name, but disappointed that they had found no cure.

A few writers have cautioned against unrealistic hopes for a cure. In 1990, for example, Dwight McGoon, a doctor who had been diagnosed with Parkinson's disease, said that "though it's important to maintain an upbeat attitude toward Parkinson's disease, let's not kid ourselves. [...] Not even the most determined patient has ever been cured or has entirely thwarted the condition's progression" (B1, p. 136). More recently, in 2013, a dozen people with Parkinson's were asked to write their answers to this question: "Will there be a cure for PD, and how soon?" Many of those who responded were skeptical. For example, Linda: "When I was first diagnosed, the doctor told me there would be a cure in five-ten years, and then I learned that everyone since has been told the same thing. [...] I don't think my generation of PwP [People with Parkinson's] will see a cure." Jackie: "I think there will be a cure but even if it were found today, it would not come to market for at least ten years because the pharma companies have no interest in curing us— not when they can make hundreds of millions of dollars off of the meds that we take." Anders: "I personally don't believe in a cure." Fulvio: "Honestly, I'm not confident I'll live long enough to see the cure for PD" (all quotations are taken from *The Peripatetic Pursuit of Parkinson Disease*, B20, pp. 285–88).

In his recent *A Parkinson's Life and a Caregiver's Roadmap* (2018), Jolyon Hallows says that even if a cure is found, it won't help his wife Sandra—or him: "Even if there is a medical breakthrough, she will still need full care. And if there isn't, she, or I, will reach the stage where I can no longer care for her, and she, or both of us, will need to move into a care home"

(p. 115). Even more recently (2019), Nick Pernisco says, "Let me make this absolutely clear: at this time, there is no cure for Parkinson's disease. There is no herb, vitamin, mineral, therapy, pill, or device that has been scientifically proven to stop, delay, or reverse the disease's progression" (p. 118).

Most doctors and patients, however, are more optimistic. They reason that if medical researchers can find a cure for bubonic plague, smallpox, polio, syphilis, and tuberculosis, surely they can find one for little old slow-moving Parkinson's. If scientists can discover how to keep people with Parkinson's moving for a while longer by giving us medications like carbidopa/levodopa, and if they can figure out how to insert electrical wires deep into our brains to keep us moving even longer, then surely it is only a matter of time until they take the next big step and find a cure for this disease. The hope for a cure is almost universal among both neurologists and their patients. The only important area of disagreement is when the cure will come. Notice the cautious references to time in the following quotations: "sometime within the next ten years," "in our lifetime," "may not be that far off," "in the pipeline," "one day":

> Tom Isaacs (2007): "It is certainly conceivable that some time within the next ten years, I might be able to insert the words 'used to' when I say, 'I have Parkinson's' " (B8, p. 330).

> Dr. Abraham Lieberman (2011): "When will there be a cure? […] I don't know, but I'm confident it'll come […] and in our lifetime" (A 13, p. 236).

> Karl Robb (2012): "For over twenty years, I have been told that in five years we are going to have a cure for Parkinson's disease. I heard this from renowned neurologists and former leaders in the Parkinson's community. They assured me that a cure was in the

pipeline. I was, and remain, skeptically hopeful" (B19, p. 262).

Dr. Sotirios A. Parashos, et al. (2013): "There is general optimism among Parkinson disease specialists that drugs that treat the disease itself, not just its symptoms, and even a cure, may not be that far off" (A15, p. 32).

Alice Lazzarini (2014): "And, because Parkinson's progresses slowly, you have every right to maintain the hope—as I do—that researchers will make further exponential progress in our lifetime. Keep the faith" (B22, p. 165).

Wendall Woodall (2014): "I'm confident that we will one day find a cure for cancer and Parkinson's and Alzheimer's and everything else that seems right now to be unbeatable. [...] Go science!" (p. 115).

Dr. Maria De León (2015): "I still believe in the promise of a better tomorrow for those who suffer many neurological illnesses like Parkinson's. The hope is to one day find a cure for Parkinson's. [...] We CAN find a CURE!" (B29, p. 12).

My own view is that there is good reason for Parkinson's patients to be cautiously hopeful about a cure. Having said that, I hasten to insist that we be careful about what we mean by "a cure for Parkinson's."

I have a hunch that a "cure," when it comes, will not fix us up like new. I do not expect that some snappy neurologist will proudly hand me a pill and say, "Take this pill, Pete, and you'll be all better by tomorrow. You'll be back the way you were two decades ago, leaping high like a gazelle, running fast like a cheetah, walking tall like a giraffe. No more stumbles or falls for you, Pete! This little pill will bring those dead cells in your substantia nigra alive again."

I anticipate that the most a "cure" might do is keep my disease from getting worse. That is, it may possibly arrest the disease in its already advanced state. I cannot imagine that it will replace the brain cells that my disease has already killed off.

I also have a hunch that when a cure does come, it will be a cure for only one or two of the many manifestations of Parkinson's. It will stop the tremors, for example, but not the freezing of gait. Or it will stop the freezing, but not the speech and voice problems.

Furthermore, I am guessing that what they will call a cure will in fact be more like a list of warnings and bits of advice: drink only distilled water; avoid all water that flows underground in agricultural parts of the country; eat no vegetables not labeled "organic"; avoid dairy products; avoid wheat products; never touch any fertilizers, pesticides, or herbicides; avoid automotive exhaust fumes; get lots of exercise; walk to work; take the stairs, not the elevator; drink nothing from a plastic bottle; eat nothing sold in a "tin" can; engage in vigorous sports rather than sitting in front of a television screen watching others engage in vigorous sports. I am guessing that the list of warnings and bits of advice will be so long and grow so fast that people will ignore it, just as many people now ignore warnings about avoiding sugar, tobacco, alcohol, narcotics, and a sedentary lifestyle.

When might such a "cure" be available for distribution to people with Parkinson's? No time soon. I fully expect that there will be a someday-cure for some kinds of Parkinson's, but not a right-away-cure for all kinds. There is no curative drug or procedure now on the horizon, let alone "in the pipeline" or "just around the corner," but even if there were, it could not get through all the tests and trials required for approval by the Food and Drug Administration in time to help most of us who have already been diagnosed. I would, of course, love to be proven wrong.

Passive hoping. As I think about how realistic it is to hope for a cure for Parkinson's, it helps me to make a distinction between passive hoping and active hoping. Hoping for a cure for Parkinson's is passive because it is hoping that someone else will discover the cure. Most of us folks with Parkinson's lack the knowledge and medical experience and the funding to design a research model, get grants, experiment with animals, seek permission to test a hypothesis in controlled, double-blind experiments on human subjects, adjust for the Hawthorne effect and the placebo effect, and so on. We must leave such research to others. We, of course, hope they succeed in finding a cure, but it is a passive hope, like hoping we will someday colonize Mars. That would be nice, we suppose, but it is not something we ourselves can make happen.

In a recent (2016) book, Terry Cason, a man with Parkinson's, tells us that it is not helpful to "sit back and anxiously hope and pray that someone comes up with a cure" (B34, p. 19). I agree. That kind of passive hoping for a cure does no one much good. I am not sure I agree, however, with what Cason says on that same page about the "good news" about Parkinson's: "The bad news is that since Parkinson's disease is progressive, our symptoms are guaranteed to get worse over time. Unfortunately, there's nothing you can do to change the direction of that course. The good news is that there's plenty you can do to prolong that journey as much as possible." I doubt that everyone with Parkinson's would necessarily agree with Cason's assumption that it is good to prolong the lives of Parkinson's patients as much as possible. Speaking here only for myself, part of what I actively hope for is not to prolong the journey—especially the end stages of the journey—as much as possible (more on that below in Chapters 15, "A Good Death,"

17, "Depression and Self-Deliverance," 19, "The ABCs of Self-Deliverance," and 20, "The Way Ahead").

Active hoping. There are lots of important things I do *actively* hope for, that is, things I can do for myself and that you can do for yourself. Here are some of the items on my own list:

I hope to do what I can to advance the search for a cure for Parkinson's, not so that I can be cured, but so that fewer people in the future will get the disease or, if they do get it, so that they will have more effective treatment options than I have had. I can, for example, volunteer for research projects that current researchers are conducting, and I can donate my posthumous brain for research study. Those actions will not help me, but they may help the next generations—and possibly my own children or grandchildren.

I hope before I die to clean out a few cluttered files, straighten up my workshop, and finish up a few writing projects—such as this one.

I hope to stand tall until I am knocked down, then get up and stand tall again until I am *really* knocked down.

I hope never to forget to be grateful for all the good things life has given me. I've been blessed by having been born into a loving family in a great nation. I had a good education, excellent job opportunities, and an enviable career.

I hope never to forget that I lucked out with an amazing wife who proved to be an amazing mother to our four amazing children and then an amazing grandmother to our nine amazing grandchildren.

I hope never to forget to be grateful that I was born in 1940 rather than in 1840. Today the average life expectancy for Americans is almost seventy-nine years. I read recently that "people with Parkinson's who do not exhibit dementia have only a one-year lower life expectancy than those who do not have the disease" (*AARP Bulletin*, March 2018, p. 22). I am seventy-nine. If I die today, I will have made it to exactly that average age. What business do I have even thinking of complaining? It helps me to remember that in 1900 the average life expectancy for Americans was only forty-seven years. If I had been born in 1840, I would probably not have lived to see a new century. I have no earthly right to complain that my dying comes too early.

I hope never to forget that I have enjoyed for three-quarters of a century near-perfect health. How dare I complain when there are billions of people on earth who have had none of the blessings I have enjoyed and who have suffered far worse health problems than I? How dare I complain that Parkinson's has limited me in my final decade, when millions of people on earth are dying of a starvation they do not deserve and bombs they did nothing to elicit? How dare I express disappointment that scientists have not found a way to cure my Parkinson's disease?

I hope to remain as self-sufficient and as independent as possible for as long as possible.

I hope that I will not burden my wife and children with a lingering or difficult end of life.

I hope to be as gracious in accepting their help as they have been in accepting my help down through the years.

I hope to leave them with memories of a strong, caring, and independent man, not of a weak, helpless, and dependent one.

I hope to convince my family, through my will and advance directives, that I do not want or intend to put myself (or them) through a long invalidism.

I hope to be able to be honest enough with myself to recognize when I am no longer having fun, learning anything new, or contributing anything to anyone.

I hope to be able to write for myself as short, as inexpensive, and as unmessy a final chapter as possible.

I hope that I will not confuse a longer life with a better life.

I hope to stay engaged in life—to enjoy people, to have goals, to be thankful—until I find a way to disengage.

I hope to be able to laugh until the end. I hope, that is, to "win" my battle with Parkinson's in the sense that Vikki Claflin talks about at the very end of her recent (2016) book: "Even without a cure in your lifetime, you can fight a good fight. There will be countless frustrations, epic fails, and a wealth of embarrassing stories to delight your offspring around the dinner table. If you can laugh, you will own that moment. And ultimately, a life made up of joyful moments means you've won" (B35, p. 201).

Dying a good death is perhaps the most realistic "cure" that those of us with late-stage Parkinson's can hope to achieve. The consequences, to ourselves and to our families, of a reluctance to consider such a cure were brought home to me by Milly in Morton Kondracke's *Saving Milly* (B2), by Scoop in Diane Rehm's *On My Own* (A27), and by Nariman in Rohinton Mistry's *Family Matters* (C4).

Read those books. You'll see what I mean.

14. The Evolution of a P-Man

[In September 2016, the fourth triannual meeting of the World Parkinson's Congress took place in Portland, Oregon. More than 4,500 people—neurologists, researchers, people with Parkinson's, care partners—from more than sixty-five countries attended. Those who registered early received a terse website invitation to submit a brief story: "The World Parkinson's Congress is looking for registrants to apply to participate in a special project at the WPC 2016 in September. To be considered for the project, please submit, in 200 words or less, the impact Parkinson's has had on your life or how your life changed because of your association to Parkinson's, whether as a researcher, clinician, or person living with it." I decided to write a series of five linked limericks. My "story" was one of the sixty-three that the editorial board accepted out of the nearly 150 submitted. When I wrote the limericks, I had been diagnosed for more than ten years. For most of those years I had a relatively easy time of it. My meds worked just fine and I got plenty of exercise walking. But then things took a rapid turn for the worse. My meds lost much of their effectiveness, I frequently experienced "freezing of gait" (FOG), and I began falling a lot. My linked limericks were published in the

World Parkinson's Congress's Faces of Parkinson's *just before Christmas, 2016.]*

At diagnosis:

So it's Parkinson's, is it? Oh, damn!
I've been hit with a full-body slam.
      My life is now done.
      There will be no more fun.
I'll go out like a wimpy, scared lamb

A few years later:

Hey, this Parkinson's strawberry jam!
It's as sweet as a marshmallowed yam.
      Yellow pills, like the sun,
      Make the shadows all run.
I'm not a scared lamb, I'm a ram!

A few years after that:

The P-word roared back with a wham!
Scared to death—that's what I now am.
      Now where can I run?
      Now where is the sun?
Park's a shark and poor Pete's just a clam.

And a couple of years after that:

I need to come up with a plan.
Is there any way out of this jam?
      I fall down when I run
      As if shot by a gun—
A disgrace to myself and my clan.

And now:

I declare on all whining a ban.
I am no wimpy lamb, ram, or clam!
      Though I stumble and tumble,
      I refuse now to grumble.
It is time Pete stood tall, like a man.

Part Two:

Dying with
Parkinson's Disease

15. A Good Death

Everyone who has Parkinson's has read or been told that "Parkinson's won't kill you. You'll die *with* Parkinson's, not *of* it." Those words are supposed to make us feel better. We are supposed to breathe a sigh of relief and say, "Oh good! Parkinson's is not fatal. It will be only a minor inconvenience." Perhaps it is just as well to let us think that—for a while.

Parkinson's is indeed for most of us just a minor inconvenience—for a while. The meds our neurologists prescribe allow us to continue our regular jobs and activities—for a while. Unless we tell them, no one even knows we have this disease—for a while.

For those who seek it, there is lots of advice available about strategies for coping in the good-time early stages of our disease: exercise, join a support group, exercise, keep a positive attitude, exercise, keep your sense of humor, exercise, take care of your care partner, and so on. But then—after a while—things are not so good anymore. Our ability to do meaningful exercise safely is reduced. Our symptoms get worse. Our neurologists run out of adjustments that work.

How we die. If people with Parkinson's do not die of

Parkinson's, how do we die? Well, we can die of cancer or heart attack or kidney failure, or stroke. We can drown in a typhoon or get bitten by a python or be stabbed by a burglar. We can get crushed in a car wreck or pulverized in a landslide or blown up by a terrorist. Since people with Parkinson's can die in all sorts of ways that have nothing to do with Parkinson's, perhaps we should rephrase the misleading statement that "Parkinson's will not kill you" and say instead that "Parkinson's will not necessarily be what kills you." And instead of telling patients, "You will die with Parkinson's, not of it," perhaps we should tell them, "You will die of Parkinson's only if you do not die of something else first."

Of course Parkinson's can kill us. To insist that people do not die of Parkinson's disease is like saying that falling off a high scaffold will not kill us—it is landing on the pavement below that does the killing. It is like saying that stepping on a land mine does not kill us—it is the loss of blood from the shredded leg arteries that does the killing.

Most of us with Parkinson's, if we do not die of some other disease or infection or mishap, will eventually die in one of three ways: from pneumonia, from complications following a fall, or from self-deliverance.

A frequent cause of death in people with Parkinson's is pneumonia. As our muscles begin to weaken, some of us have trouble swallowing. As a result, we sometimes "aspirate" particles of food or drops of liquid—that is, suck them down the windpipe into the lungs. We try to cough them up, but as our Parkinson's progresses, we lack the strength to cough vigorously enough to expel fully the food or liquids, and they tend to remain and fester in our lungs. The result can be an infection known as pneumonia, which is sometimes called "the old man's friend" because it can lead, if untreated, to a straightforward and gentle dying.

Another cause of death for people with Parkinson's is falling. It is common knowledge that Parkinson's often affects our balance. We "freeze" or stumble or trip. Surprisingly, relatively few of us who fall will die from a head injury. More likely to cause death is a fall resulting in broken bones that leads to hospitalization or surgery. Surgery introduces the possibility of infection. Furthermore, surgery often limits or prevents normal exercise during and after recovery. Reduced physical activity is never good, but it is especially risky for people who have Parkinson's. Hip fractures are especially dangerous for us and often lead to death.

A third reasonably common death option for people with Parkinson's is "self-deliverance"—a term that some people find less offensive than "suicide," though they don't so much mind using the latter term if it is modified by "assisted." See, for example, the subtitle of Derek Humphry's *Final Exit: The Practicalities of Self-Deliverance and Assisted Suicide for the Dying* (2002). Some writers prefer the term "assisted death" to the term "assisted suicide."

It is not easy to find reliable advice about how to deal with the later stages of Parkinson's: the years when we can no longer walk through the door to a support group meeting, let alone drive to the disabled parking spot just outside that door; the years when we choke on the meds we take to keep us from choking; the years when we can no longer wipe ourselves, bathe ourselves, or dress ourselves, let alone do push-ups, chin-ups, sit-ups, or even stand-ups; the years when we can find less to laugh at and fewer to laugh with; the years when we can think of nothing we can do to help our care partners except hope that they won't have to take care of us for too much longer.

Many writers have written about death and dying. Few have felt inclined to explore the reality of a Parkinson's death. Those who know about that reality don't want to write about it because it is not a pretty picture. They want to protect us from the truths that they fear—with some justification—may only discourage us even further. Those who are dying generally cannot write about it because they are immobilized, exhausted, or confused—

perhaps all three. They merely want to get on with their dying.

To give you some notion of what a Parkinson's death can be like, I want to introduce you to two women. They never met, never even heard of each other, but they came to share similar views about death and dying. One is my mother, Margaret Grant Beidler. The other is a palliative care nurse named Sallie Tisdale.

Mother. Margaret Grant was born in Houghton, Michigan, in 1909. I never met her father, Elmer Grant, who died in 1935, five years before I was born. He took a job as a mathematics professor at Earlham College in Richmond, Indiana, and Margaret eventually attended Earlham, majoring in English. Soon after she graduated, she left for Ramallah, Jordan, to teach English at a Quaker school there. On the ship sailing across the Atlantic Ocean and the Mediterranean Sea, she met Paul Beidler, a handsome young archaeologist on his way to Iraq to help excavate an ancient site there.

Five years later, after Paul finished his degree in architecture at the University of Pennsylvania, they married and started a family. Born in 1940, I was the third of their four children and only son.

The marriage was rocky, but it lasted, more or less, until the late 1950s. By then my father was working as a foreign service officer in Phnom Penh, Cambodia, and my mother was teaching English to Buddhist monks at a temple there. Meanwhile, we got word that my mother's mother, Josephine Grant, was becoming senile and would soon need to be placed in an institution. My mother decided she needed to return to Indiana to look after her mother. By then my two older sisters, Jo and Sue, had finished high school and were about to start their own independent lives, Jo as a draftsman, Sue as a nurse. My younger sister Fran and I went with Mother to help with Grandma Jo and finish high school. My father stayed in Phnom Penh.

Grandma Jo died a year later. My parents decided that

Mother, Fran, and I should stay in Richmond for another year so I could finish high school and Mother could attend to legal matters relating to Grandma Jo's belongings and estate. I assumed that at the end of that year my mother would pack her bags and head back to wifehood in Phnom Penh, but by then my parents had noticed that they were both happier apart than together. They decided that it might be just as well for Mother to stay in Richmond, where she had been offered a good job as executive secretary to the president of Earlham College.

My parents eventually divorced. Paul stayed in Asia until he retired, then brought back with him a young Thai woman as his bride. Down through the years, Mother had a number of teaching, counseling, and executive jobs in various parts of the country. Then she retired and moved to a delightful retirement community a couple of hours north of Los Angeles, where my younger sister Fran lived.

Mother had a happy dozen or so years in her little bungalow in the retirement community. I visited her there at least once a year. She took one meal a day in the dining room. She and Mary, her best friend, loved walking along the beach near a little seaside restaurant called the Brown Pelican. Whenever we visited, Mother took my sister Fran and me there for breakfast. She always recited her favorite limerick:

> What a wonderful bird is the Pelican.
> His mouth can hold more than his belly can.
> > He can hold in his beak
> > Enough food for a week,
> But I don't see how in the hell he can.

Mother died in the infirmary of that retirement community. She was never diagnosed with Parkinson's, but I am pretty sure—now that I am familiar with the symptoms—that she had it. She froze in doorways. She stumbled and fell several times. She had a wandering pinky-finger on her left hand and could no longer type. She tended to shuffle when she walked.

She had lived independently in her own lovely bungalow on the premises of the retirement community for that dozen years, but as she grew older, the demands of daily living became more and more difficult. She decided at age eighty-nine that she would give up her beloved bungalow and move into a shared assisted-living apartment in the same retirement community.

Mother was not happy about the change: "Do I really want to make this move? Do I really want to trade my independence and my bungalow for dependence and the right to share a living room with three other sick old ladies?" Her unstated answer to both questions was clearly "No," but she also recognized that, as she put it: "It is time." People who live in retirement communities hear death knocking on doors all around them. Mother and her friends found themselves asking, when they learned that someone they knew had died, "Was it a good death?"

A good death. For them, a good death was one that was quick, unexpected, and without pain, mess, or expensive fuss. It usually meant a death that came when one was old, but not *too* old, when one was still able to live mostly independently, when one still "had their wits about them." A good death left your friends saying, "Oh, good. It is just what she wanted! It was time. It was quick."

Just a couple of weeks before Mother was to move to assisted living, she was having lunch with several of her good friends when they noticed she was acting a little strange. Her best friend, Mary, suggested that the two of them take a little walk over to the infirmary to check things out. Mother angrily refused. Another of her friends excused herself and called the infirmary to tell the supervisor about Mother's unusual behavior. The supervisor said she would come right over with a wheelchair. Mother protested again, but let them take her. It turned out that she had just had a stroke, a pretty bad one.

Mother never got to return to her bungalow, never moved

to her shared assisted living unit. She was given a bed in the infirmary.

The supervisor called my sister Fran, whom Mother had designated as her durable power of attorney for health care decisions. When Fran arrived, she found Mother all but unconscious in the hospital bed. Fran could speak to her but not with her because Mother was not able to speak. Fran called me and I caught the next plane from Pennsylvania. Together we talked with Mother's doctor, who told us that the staff of the infirmary would be able to feed and hydrate our mother, but that her stroke was a bad one. She would almost certainly not recover in any meaningful sense of the word.

Fran and I called our other two sisters (Jo, in Pennsylvania, and Sue—a nurse—in Australia). We all agreed that Mother had let us know in various ways over the years that she did not want to be kept alive in such a situation, that she had had a good, long life and was not afraid of dying. She had filed an advance directive with her doctor, who told us what our options were. One of the options was tube feeding, which we knew Mother did not want. The option we took was that the nursing staff would place a plate of food and a glass of water on the table beside Mother's bed but would not spoon-feed her or hold the glass to her lips. If she reached for the food or the glass, fine, but if not—well, they would keep her comfortable.

What did Mother die of? Did she die of Parkinson's? Probably not, since she was never diagnosed with the disease. Did she die of a stroke? Well, not really, because she technically survived that first stroke and then a second, smaller one a few days later. Did we four children murder her? Well, not really, because we all knew she wanted no part of tube-fed or nurse-fed nourishment. Was her death a suicide? Probably not, since she did not move that day to take her own life. She left no suicide note—unless we consider the advance directive to be one. She pulled no trigger, leapt off no cliff, flashed no razor, swallowed no pill, dangled no rope, tied no plastic bag. On her death certificate, the doctor wrote down as the cause of death "renal failure," but was that renal failure really more an effect of her starvation and dehydration than the cause of her death? Ambiguity often reigns in the kingdom of the dying.

For Mother herself, the important question would have been not "What did she die of?" but "Was it a good death?" I think she and her friends would have thought Mother's was a pretty good death. It was time. She was old, but not *too* old. She still had her wits about her. She was spared the move to assisted living. Her death was quick enough, unexpected enough, and as deaths go, not painful, messy, or expensive.

Tisdale. A woman named Sallie Tisdale worked for many years as a palliative care nurse in an intensive care unit (ICU). Her job was to keep the patients sent to her alive as long as possible, whether or not they wanted to be kept alive. She came to believe that it was wrong to assume that anyone who was dying ought to be rescued from death. She devotes a whole chapter of her recent (2018) book, *Advice for Future Corpses,* to "A Good Death." She tells us that most people define a good death as "one free of pain, peaceful and calm." A good death includes family and friends, and a chance to reflect on one's life" (p. 39). Tisdale argues that, based on her experience as a palliative care nurse, most actual deaths, even though they bear little resemblance to these romanticized notions, are in fact good deaths. She questions whether fighting death can really contribute to a good death. She says this about cardio-pulmonary resuscitation: "I do believe that CPR, like all kinds of supposedly life-supporting treatments, interferes with a peaceful death. [...] Is it possible to have a good death in the midst of desperately trying to stay alive?" (p. 59).

Die at home or in a hospital? My mother's actual death took place not in her bungalow with her family gathered around her bed offering testimonials of love and attending tearfully to her dying words of wisdom, reconciliation, love, whatever. If that is the kind of death she envisioned or wanted, she never told Fran or me about it. I am guessing that she did not want that. If so, why move to a retirement community with an infirmary? I think she moved there in part because she wanted her death to be presided over by people who knew what they were doing.

If we have strong feelings about where we want to die, we should of course let that be known. It is easy to announce to your family that you want to die at home and not in some expensive impersonal hospital or nursing home under the care of paid strangers. But even so simple a decision as that is easily complicated by a disease like Parkinson's. Is it really fair for you to decide that you want to die at home without considering whether such a request assumes that your family is willing and able to look after you there—perhaps for a long, long time?

Tisdale's book is not specifically about Parkinson's, but she speaks briefly about her personal experience with one man with the disease:

> I sometimes see a sixty-two-year-old man with rapidly progressive Parkinson's disease. He is in the last months of his life now. He has trouble swallowing, and the disease has caused painful contractures and akathisia: he is constantly restless and agitated; his body can't stop moving. He pedals and kicks and stretches and sits up and lies down. He says to me in what remains of his whispering voice, "I'm done with all this. There's no point in living." (p. 91)

Drawing on many years of experience as a hospice and palliative care nurse, Tisdale urges that we be realistic about what dying at home can involve. It is easy to imagine our beloved aging relative reclining in his own bed wearing the flannel pajamas his wife Irma had made for him last Christmas. It is easy to imagine Irma bringing in a platter of his favorite meal—meatloaf and mashed potatoes smothered in gravy. It is easy to imagine his daughter bringing her two sons in to play one last game of Hearts with their grandfather before she trundles them off to bed, this being a school night. It is easy to imagine the dying man whispering, "I love you, Irma," as he slips away into his long final sleep. No wonder we want to die at home being taken care of by people who know and love us.

But that happy scenario rarely matches the reality of an actual dying scenario.

Today, most Americans do not die at home. Eighty percent of us die in a hospital or nursing home. Tisdale puts it this way:

> The amount of what is known as "bedside care" required by a dying patient is more than a challenge to untrained caregivers. How will you handle confusion or agitation in the middle of the night? What will you do if a person falls? What happens if there is bleeding? Can you change the clothing or the bed linens if a person throws up or has diarrhea? Are you prepared to stay awake all night? (p. 95)

Tisdale offers wise counsel when she writes:

> [Grandpa] may actually want the professional attention, twenty-four-hour care, and security that a hospital provides. [...] Hospitals are controlled environments and may feel safer to a fragile person than a house at the end of a long road or an apartment in a large complex of strangers. You can have a bad death in your own bed and a good death in an ICU. (pp. 93 –94)
>
> Cost is also an important consideration:
>
> Depending on your insurance coverage, your status with Medicare or Medicaid, and your specific personal finances, it may be that you cannot afford anything but dying at home—if you even have a home.

Michael Hebb, in his 2018 book, *Let's Talk About Death,* reminds us that dying can easily wipe us out financially:

> A study from the Mt. Sinai School of Medicine found that 43 percent of Medicare recipients spend more than their total assets—out of pocket—on end-of-life care. Medical care is the number one factor in US bankruptcies, with end-of-life care expenses—particularly hospital expenses—leading the charges. […] People are bankrupting their families, and for little good reason: most of them don't even want expensive, extreme life-prolonging measures, but they haven't talked to their families about their preferences, and no one has asked. (p. 7)

Each Parkinson's patient's financial situation and medical insurance situation is different, of course, just as each Parkinson's patient's disease progression and death are different. You should consider all these differences as you discuss your hopes and plans with key members of your family, your legal and financial advisers, and your medical teams: "If you don't talk about what you want at the end, then you can be sure that you won't get what you want" (p. 11).

Over my dead body. What do you want done with what is left of your earthly remains after you die? My mother wrote a poem about that when she was in her thirties:

Instructions for Burial
    by Margaret Beidler

When I am done with this
Let it return soon
To the cycle of creation.
Do not detain it from its allotted part
In the ever-nibbling growth of being.

Restrain with neither stony vault
Nor coffin wall nor wrapping shroud.

Lay it in warm moist earth
And cover it. Then let the quiet
Ceaseless processes of life reclaim it
Again from death.

Perhaps it will nourish grass
To tempt the newborn stiff-legged lamb
Whose later wool and meat will
Warm and feed some human things.

Or through the grubbing worm,
Who knows, it may arise on soaring wings—

Life is too great a miracle to miss.
Let it return, when I am done with this.

Mother knew we could not legally bury her in "in warm soft earth," though it is interesting that we could now, through Seattle's recently approved "Recompose" program and the excited talk about "green burials."

Tisdale never met my mother, but they would surely have agreed about the indecency of embalming. Tisdale disdainfully refers to embalming as a totally unnecessary rip-off and as "the art of complete denial" (p. 162). Tisdale talks about the possibility of a truly "natural burial" and the composting of human bodies: "The idea of knowing that I could become compost, could be truly used after death, is deeply satisfying" (p. 174). I think my mother and Sallie Tisdale would have liked each other.

After she moved to California, Mother altered her request

for burial without a coffin. "I have revised my thinking," she wrote, "and have arranged for cremation and burial at sea." My sister Fran and I accompanied the little fishing boat she had paid for in advance. It is perfectly legal in California to scatter human ashes in the Pacific Ocean so long as you go three miles offshore. We asked the captain of the little charter fishing boat to take us out across from the Brown Pelican. When he got more or less there, he cut the engine. He listened respectfully as we read some of Mother's poems aloud. We read "Instructions for Burial" of course. Then I read a sonnet I had written when I was a student at Earlham College in the late 1960s:

Advertisement for a Mortuary
by Peter G. Beidler

First we open up your still-warm veins
And pump that other lasting fluid through,
Then coat your face with pastel powdered stains
To give your friends a reassuring view.
Next, tenderly, we take your Sunday suit
And slit it down the back (for otherwise
We could not get your stiffened self into it).
In whitest shirt and most discreet of ties
We lay you gently in your satined coffin,
Touch up your final face and comb your hair;
The stuffy air with lily scents we soften
And play sweet music to you lying there.
We undertake with soft upholstering art
To soothe the shock of stillness in your heart.

Finally, we read Mother's wonderfully wise and hopeful poem equating the portal of birth to the portal of death:

The Portal
by Margaret Beidler

Is death a wall
Or unlocked door
To space we could not use before?

I died once.
So did you.
Expelled from all the life we knew.
Torn from the warm
Enfolding womb,
Outcast, our rage became a scream,
But with that shocked
Dismay at death
Our untried lungs found air … and breath.

Then we scattered Mother's ashes and tossed a bouquet of
red roses—one by one—into the peaceful Pacific swells.

After we got back to the marina, we drove the short distance
north to the Brown Pelican and had a late breakfast. It wasn't
quite the same without Mother there, but we knew she was not
far away.

A good death?

Yes.

16. Power of Attorney and Advance Directive

ONE OF THE REASONS WHY MY mother died a good death is that she had officially designated my sister Fran as her durable power of attorney for health care decisions. Another is that she had filed an advance directive with her doctor and the infirmary in the retirement community she called home. In this chapter I want to say a little more about each of those important steps.

I am sure you know that you should ask a lawyer who understands the inheritance laws of your state to prepare a will naming a power of attorney for financial and legal matters. That person may well also be named as executor of your estate after your death. It is also advisable for you to take two other actions to prepare the way for the kind of death you want and the kind of dying you hope for.

1. Designate a durable power of attorney for health care decisions. This is the first and most important step. Discuss the matter with a lawyer. My mother designated my sister Fran, who lived only two hours away in Los Angeles, as her health care power of attorney. Typically, the person named is a spouse or a blood relative, preferably one who lives nearby. There may well come a time when Parkinson's patients need assistance with their health care or need counsel on key decisions about housing, treatments, and end-of-life options.

The person best positioned to fill such a role is usually assumed to be the spouse, partner, or child of the patient. You should, of course, make sure they are willing to serve as your "agent" if and when it becomes necessary. If they agree, that agreement should be spelled out in a legal document signed well in advance of the time such an agent is needed. It is also good to have alternate names on file in case the first person named is unavailable. I have designated my wife Anne as my agent or durable power of attorney for health care decisions, and I designate our four children as alternates. Similarly, in her document, Anne designates me as her power of attorney for health care decisions, with our four children listed as alternates.

A power of attorney document stipulates the person who will speak for you and make all decisions regarding your health care, treatment, and the professionals who treat you once you are no longer able to speak for yourself. Your designated agent can say yes or no to treatments or surgery, decide where you will go for treatment and care, decide whether you need certain medications or procedures, decide when these are no longer working and enough is enough. Because every state has different rules regarding what is permitted as we near the end of our lives, it is important that you seek out professional advice that applies in your state regarding this directive. For instance, Washington passed a Death with Dignity Act; most other states have not.

In addition to designating your power of attorney for health care decisions, you should provide an "advance directive" informing your agent, your family, and key members of your medical team about your end-of-life preferences.

2. Write an advance directive in which you let your doctors, family, and designated power of attorney for health care decisions know your wishes about end-of-life issues. The document must be signed, dated, and witnessed. The life-and-death decisions that lie ahead will be based on this statement of your preferences about end-of-life issues like resuscitation, feeding tubes, mechanical breathing pumps, and intravenous hydration. If you do not have such a document, made when you are clear-headed and thinking logically about such things, decisions may be made for you that are against your wishes. With no such advance directive to guide them, health care workers must assume that the longest possible life is what you want, no matter what the cost, the prognosis, or the likely benefit.

There is much to be gained by issuing an advance directive. It will give you peace of mind to let others know your wishes for the future. You can always change your mind later on. The following is a summary of my directive, meaning that it expresses my wishes. These may not be yours.

In this directive, I am letting my family and friends know I prefer a "natural death" when it is determined that further measures will only prolong the dying process because my condition is "incurable and irreversible" with "no reasonable possibility of recovery." This directive gives clear permission to stop medical and surgical treatment when it is no longer working and assures everyone concerned that these are my express wishes and that under these circumstances, I do not wish to be given any food or drink that must be administered artificially. If it is confirmed by my physician to the satisfaction of my agent that I have dementia, whatever I say to the contrary of this directive should be ignored. My agent is instructed to have me moved to a facility where my needs will be met and where I will be kept comfortable and pain-free. Once my dementia is moderate to severe, I do not wish to receive medical treatment that will prolong my life unnaturally. As for the treatment of pain, my agent will determine what medications or treatments are necessary, even if they are unconventional, damage me further physically, and unintentionally hasten my death. After I am dead, my body will benefit medical research and my organs will be available for transplant. Finally, I proclaim that I am "emotionally and mentally" capable of approving this directive and can alter or delete language at any time if I change my mind regarding any of its stipulations.

I do not, of course, expect that your advance directive will resemble mine. It should, rather, reflect your own wishes and expectations. It is best if your advance directive is made in consultation with key members of your family.

On May 18, 2019, Daniel Low, a family medicine resident at a Seattle hospital, published in the *Seattle Times* a short personal essay titled, "Why won't we talk about death?" In the article he argued that we should all have honest "conversations" with members of our family to let them know our thoughts and feelings about end-of-life issues. He mentioned having witnessed a ninety-five-year-old man whose ribs were "crushed and crumpled like papier-mâché during CPR because there was no documentation indicating he wanted anything differently." Dr. Low said that a month before that he had sat anxiously with a family "trying to decide whether to 'pull the plug' on their comatose father/husband, uncertain of his wishes, having never had that conversation." Dr. Low went on:

> Many of us live in denial about death—shying away from discussing it. Many medical professionals act as if death is a problem to be solved, rather than a process to be lived. Consequently, while 92% of people believe talking with their loved ones about end-of-life care is important, only 32% of people do so. Similarly, while 97% of people say it is important to put their wishes in writing, only 37% of people have such written documentation.

I suggest that you take the lead in starting the necessary conversations. Your doctor will feel awkward about raising the subject unless you are about to undergo a risky operation.

Members of your family will feel awkward about raising the subject for fear that you will assume they think you are about to die or even that they want you to die so they can get their hands on their inheritance. No, you should take charge, gather key members of your family together, and start the conversation. You might say, for example: "Thanks for coming over. I've been thinking that it is not too early to share with you my thoughts about certain end-of-life issues. We all know that one of these days I am going to take a bad fall. You will perhaps need to make some important life-and-death decisions. I want you all to take a look at a draft of the advance directive that will let you and my doctors know I want to be allowed to die a natural death. I do not want to be given CPR or fed intravenously or put on any sort of life-support machine. I ask that you honor my wishes and direct hospice people to keep me comfortably sedated during my dying time. Whether I die at home or in a nursing home or hospital does not matter to me. At home is probably cheaper, unless Medicare will cover the cost of a nursing home. Do you have any questions, suggestions, or concerns?"

Having this conversation with key members of your family will give them a chance to understand what you want and to clarify your decisions. It will save them the agony of someday trying to guess what you might have preferred. Having given copies of the document to key members of your family and your health care team, you can rest easy knowing you have taken the vital first steps toward taking charge of your own end-of-life planning. You have given to another person the authority to insist that your wishes are honored by medical staff and you have expressed your thoughts about artificially prolonging your life as opposed to being permitted to die a natural death.

You have taken charge. Well done, boss!

17. Depression and Self-Deliverance

I WANT TO EMPHASIZE HERE AT THE start of this chapter that I do not wish to be misread as an advocate for suicide. If you think you know someone who is contemplating suicide, please intervene and suggest that they call the National Suicide Prevention Lifeline at 1-800-273-8255. If the person you are concerned about is older than sixty, you can suggest that they call 1-800-971-0016, the Friendship Line at the Institute on Aging.

The people I am addressing in this chapter are the men and women who are in the last stages of a neurodegenerative, progressive, and incurable disease like Parkinson's. These are men and women who have tried everything their doctors have suggested, but even so find themselves slipping into a life of useless inactivity, a life of total dependency, a life of wheelchairs and bedside commodes, a life requiring assistance in toileting, dressing, bathing, and eating. I am addressing the men and women who have tried everything and who know that their disease will soon make them totally dependent on others for their most fundamental and personal needs. For such people, the term "suicide" seems particularly inappropriate. It is too harsh, too naked, too strong, too wrong.

Most people seem to associate suicide with unhappiness, failure, or depression. We think of it as a secret, lonely, desperate, violent, and messy act done by someone who is young or in generally good health. We think of Hamlet's suicidal lament that God had forbidden "self-slaughter." We think of Julius Caesar's falling on his sword or Cleopatra's holding an asp to her breast. We think of Madame Bovary's swallowing arsenic or Ernest Hemingway's blowing his brains out by toeing the trigger of a shotgun. We think of Willy Loman's driving his car into a bridge abutment or Thelma and Louise driving their convertible off a cliff. We think of Robin Williams, not long after he was diagnosed with Parkinson's, noosing himself in his bedroom.

Killing oneself, however, is not always so violent and messy. We have developed language that suggests distinctions. "Suicide attack" sounds either better or worse than plain "suicide." It sounds better if it involves a military hero protecting his fellow soldiers by charging into an enemy bunker with a live hand grenade. It sounds worse if it involves a terrorist hijacking and crashing a domestic passenger plane into an office building. The term "suicide" usually sounds better when it is accompanied by another word, as in "attempted suicide," "assisted suicide," "rational suicide," or "suicide mission." "Assisted suicide" sounds less brutal than plain "suicide," if only because the death is a somewhat social act, not a solitary one. "Rational suicide" sounds more reasonable than plain "suicide" because the qualifying term suggests that the person thinking of killing him- or herself has thought about it carefully and is not acting out of irrational despair or impulsive depression. I first encountered the term "rational suicide" in a June 24, 2019, *Seattle Times* article by Melissa Bailey under the headline "Some Seniors Considering Options of 'Rational Suicide.' " The opening paragraph of the article reads:

Ten residents slipped away from their retirement

community one Sunday afternoon for a covert meeting in a grocery-store café. They aimed to answer a taboo question: When they feel they have lived long enough, how can they carry out their own swift and peaceful death?

We have developed a series of euphemisms to soften the blow of suicide: "taking one's own life," "doing oneself in," "graceful exit," "finding peace," "elective death," "death with dignity," "going to a better place," "compassionate choice," "carrying out one's own swift and peaceful death." "Self-deliverance" has gained some traction because it sounds both more civilized and less violent than "self-destruction," "self-slaughter," and "self-murder." The term "self-deliverance," then, might be called a gentle euphemism for "suicide" by suggesting that a person acts not out of depression or sudden impulse but after having thought carefully about the alternatives. It also suggests rescue or escape, as in the familiar expressions "deliver us from temptation" and "deliver us from evil." The term suggests that the person does not disappear into an abyss but rather gets "delivered" to some specific and meaningful destination—kind of like an Amazon package, complete with the smile on the cardboard.

Are there justifiable reasons for a Parkinson's self-deliverance? For some of us, the answer to that question is unequivocal: "There are no justifiable reasons." We have been told that it is flat-out wrong to take our own lives. We have been told that to commit suicide—by whatever name—is pridefully to claim as our own a decision that should be left to God. We have been told that suicide is a coward's way to escape our responsibilities. We have been told that suicide harms others who are left with guilt for not having seen the signs and prevented it. We have been told that suicide is caused by depression and that any person who contemplates suicide ought to seek counseling and antidepressant medications. We have been told that suicide usually leaves to others the familial, legal, financial, and biological messes that the dead person has selfishly escaped. We have been told that suicide is a nasty way to take revenge against someone who has hurt or angered us. We have been told that suicide makes a selfish mockery of love.

Suicide can, of course, be all of those things and worse— particularly if the attempt is botched and the person is left alive but even more wounded, angry, frightened, and pathetically dependent.

But for some of us, to be refused the solace of choice about matters of our own life and death seems to condemn us to a life of senseless suffering, pricey poverty, demeaning dependence, and messy misery. For some of us, self-deliverance can be an attractive alternative to extending the worst features of Parkinson's: the dementia, the immobility, the lack of productivity, the dependence on others, the expense, and the guilt of knowing that we are subtracting from the lives and financial resources of the people we care most deeply about.

We are aware that we did nothing knowingly to bring on our Parkinson's. Was it a mysterious genetic aberration we inherited? Was it growing up in a rural community and drinking well water tainted by herbicides? Was it being drafted and sent to Vietnam, where we were ordered to live in the vicinity of a wonder-weapon called Agent Orange? Was it taking a job in a dry-cleaning establishment where we had daily contact with harsh chemicals and fumes? Was it using a certain kind of fertilizer on our garden, a certain kind of weed killer on the edges of our driveway, or a certain kind of bugspray on our fruit trees? Most of us will never know for sure. By the time we begin to show symptoms of the disease that now has us contemplating an early deliverance from a life of undignified and demeaning dependence, it is too late to go back and avoid whatever it was that brought it on. We know that we cannot prevent this disease from negatively affecting our own lives, but there are some steps we can take to minimize the negative effects on the lives, patience, and resources of the care partners and family members who have already given so much to our disease.

"Are you depressed?" My neurologist asked me that question this past spring (2018). It was near the end of one our regular three-month-interval sessions. "Your meds don't seem to be helping as much as they used to. Your exercise is down. You are falling with some regularity. You have trouble sleeping. You are constipated. You seem discouraged. It is common for people who have Parkinson's to be depressed."

"I don't think I am depressed," I said. "I love life. I am busy reading and writing. I am looking forward, with Anne, to attending our son Paul's wedding. I'm going deep-sea fishing in our son Kurt's new boat, *Sane Asylum*. Anne and I are visiting our daughter Calloway on Prince Edward Island, out in the Atlantic Maritimes. And we will be rooting for our daughter Nora's son's basketball team. I work at my writing every day. Sure, I get frustrated that my Parkinson's slows me down so much and makes me dependent on Anne and others. I get exasperated when I realize that most people cannot understand me when I try to speak. I get discouraged when I see evidence that my meds are less effective than they used to be. I get scared when I keep falling down all the time. But I don't feel depressed."

"There are things," she went on, "that we can do about depression. But before we talk antidepressants, I'd like you to talk with the social worker we have on staff here. Okay? She will give you a short mood-assessment test and talk with you about what it reveals."

The following week I visited the social worker. She handed me a sheet of paper with ten multiple-choice questions. "Don't try to analyze the questions," she said. "Just check the boxes that best fit your feelings in the past couple of weeks."

I filled out the one-page pencil-and-paper questionnaire. I

don't have a copy of the test, but the questions were all in this pattern:

1. How often have you been bothered by feeling down or hopeless over the last two weeks?
[   ] NOT AT ALL
[   ] SEVERAL DAYS
[   ] MORE THAN HALF THE DAYS
[   ] NEARLY EVERY DAY

2. How often have you been bothered by feeling anxious or on edge over the last two weeks?
[   ] NOT AT ALL
[   ] SEVERAL DAYS
[   ] MORE THAN HALF THE DAYS
[   ] NEARLY EVERY DAY

I checked NOT AT ALL on most of the questions. The last question was different:

10. How often have you thought about taking your own life in the last two weeks?
[   ] NOT AT ALL
[   ] SEVERAL DAYS
[   ] MORE THAN HALF THE DAYS
[   ] NEARLY EVERY DAY

On that last one I checked NEARLY EVERY DAY and wrote in the margin, "but that is because I have Parkinson's, not because I am depressed. I am trying to be realistic about the nasty-slow death that comes with this disease. It is not so much that I want to kill myself as that I don't want to wait around— and force the people I love most to wait around with me—for that kind of nasty-slow death."

The social worker looked at my answers, smiled, and asked me to explain my answer to the tenth question.

"I'll try," I said, "but I am not sure I can say anything more than the obvious. I wish I did not have Parkinson's, but I have it. I know that if allowed to run its usual course, Parkinson's will take me out the long, slow way. I find that way to be unappealing, but that does not mean I am depressed. I don't feel depressed, at least not in the usual sense of that term. It seems that most people, when they think about depression, think of taking antidepressants. I don't want them. I want to try to march boldly into the future, face forward."

"I think I understand," she said. "You want to spare yourself and your family the agony and expense that you think lies ahead. Is that right?"

"Yes, but that does not mean I am depressed, does it? Look. I am seventy-eight. I've had a charmed life. The thought of being dead is not unpleasant. The thought of a long, drawn-out, disabled dying is worse than unpleasant—it is abhorrent. Sure, I think about doing myself in someday, but that does not mean I am suicidal, does it? I am thinking about future options, not present actions."

"It's fine with me not to call you either depressed or suicidal," she replied. "And while antidepressants might lighten your load somewhat, they won't change the basic facts of your disease or make you abhor becoming a burden to others any less. You know, my father was diagnosed with Parkinson's last year, and he too hates to be labeled. Like you, he seems to worry about becoming a burden to Mom and me. We tell him we want him not to think anymore about that 'burden' nonsense, but I know he does. Tell me, have you made any specific preparations or inquiries about ways to end your life? I mean, have you gathered supplies that you might eventually use?"

"Not really," I said. I told her I had made some preliminary inquiries about renting helium tanks used to blow up party balloons, but that seemed too complicated. I told her that I had bought a flexible hose that could fit over the tailpipe on my Suburban and have it enter the cab through a rust hole in the back fender, but soon after that I stopped driving and gave the Suburban away. I said I had thought about a plastic bag but had not purchased the turkey-roasting bag or the bungee cords I would need.

"How does your wife feel about this?"

"Anne doesn't like it, of course, but she knows how stubborn I can be. And she knows I want to spare her the grim task of taking care of me when I get bedridden."

"Have you thought what a shock it would be for her to come home and find you dead on the floor with a turkey-roasting plastic bag over your head?"

"I have," I said. "I don't want to do that to her, but I like that better than the thought of her having to dress me, feed me, empty my bedpans or my bedside commode, and bathe my living but lifeless body for the next several miserable years."

"Have you heard," she said, "about something called Voluntarily Stopping Eating and Drinking? It is usually referred to by the initials V-S-E-D? It is pronounced VEE-said."

"I think so. But if it involves voluntarily stopping eating and drinking, it sounds like a miserable death—sort of like wandering for days in the desert looking for a rabid gopher to eat or a shriveled cactus to drink. Do you recommend this VSED thing?"

"Absolutely not! But if you are determined to consider the options, this is one you might investigate. You can read about it on the End of Life Washington website."

"Okay, thanks."

Not long after that meeting I read Sallie Tisdale's *Advice for Future Corpses*. I was pleased to read what Tisdale said about the distinction between feeling depressed and feeling demoralized:

Depression can be caused by medications or

organic changes in the brain. Many signs of a clinical depression—withdrawal from social relationships, losing interest in typical activities, talking less, eating less, sleeping more, and so on—look a lot like the late stages of dying. The experience we call demoralization can arise out of a sense of meaninglessness, a loss of purpose, or deep spiritual distress. A person can be demoralized without being depressed. This moment may be tolerable or even happy, but illness and physical decline is such a loss that the person sees no meaningful future ahead. A young person with ALS might be in this state; alive now, happy to be alive now, but starkly aware of the future to come. This isn't depression; it's a kind of bleak, honest appraisal of reality. (pp. 90–91)

Happy to be alive now, but starkly aware of what is to come, a kind of bleak, honest appraisal of reality. Sounds like Parkinson Pete.

18. Starvation and Dehydration

E ND OF LIFE WASHINGTON, ONCE KNOWN as the Hemlock
Society, is dedicated to letting people know why, when,
where, and how to self-deliver. On their website I found this
description of VSED:

Voluntarily Stopping Eating and Drinking (VSED)

When people die naturally of diseases such as cancer,
they often lose their appetites and eventually stop
eating altogether. Some people hasten the dying process
the same way, by VSED. If a person stops eating and
drinking, death may come as early as a few days, but
more commonly one to three weeks. It is especially
important to avoid sips of water or other liquids, as this
may prolong the process. A person who begins VSED
prior to its natural occurrence should expect hunger
and thirst for a few days, so it is very important to have
swabs for dry mouth and reliable access to medication to
decrease or eliminate symptoms. When done properly,
VSED usually results in a peaceful, humane death, and
many people have used this method successfully. End
of Life Washington recommends that people choosing

VSED discuss their decision with family members, caregivers, and involved medical providers to prevent them from undermining the process by offering or encouraging the intake of food or water. Make sure they are knowledgeable in helping people use VSED. End of Life Washington believes that hospice or palliative care is essential during VSED. Under some circumstances, VSED may also be utilized to hasten death for individuals who have an incurable, progressive illness which is eventually terminal, but not within the six months required for the Death with Dignity Act. Examples are illnesses such as Parkinson's, MS, other neurological diseases, and the early stages of dementia when the person is still legally competent.

I noted the specific mention of Parkinson's in the last sentence. The End of Life Washington website lists a number of frequently asked questions about VSED and gives answers. I quote a few of these here:

a. Do I need to be terminal (meaning death within six months is expected)? No.

b. Do I need my physician's permission to begin VSED? No. You do not need a physician's permission, but it is very important to have a physician support you during the process by prescribing medication for pain and anxiety, if needed. Ask your physician to refer you to hospice during the process.

c. I don't like the idea of not drinking. Can't I just stop eating? A person can live a very long time without eating, but dehydration (lack of fluids) is what speeds up the process. Dying from lack of food alone can be more prolonged and uncomfortable than dying from dehydration.

d. It seems like this would take a lot of will power.

Does it? It takes some determination, but we often find that people who make this choice are ready to "let go" and are able to be successful.

e. What about my friends and family? What will this be like for them? We suggest that you talk with your close family members and friends early about your wishes and why you want to take this course.

f. What kind of help will I need? You cannot do this alone. You will need the care of friends, family, or other caregivers during this process. If you reside in a care facility, you will need the agreement of the staff to provide support and assistance. Your physician is very important. Talk with him or her and make sure appropriate medication will be available to keep you comfortable. Ask your physician for a referral to a local hospice provider.

g. What should I do before I start? State in writing the circumstances under which it is your intention to stop eating and drinking to hasten your death. Clearly state that you want no food or fluids either by mouth, IV, or feeding tube.

I asked around about VSED. My friend Griggs reminded me that there is a chapter titled "Self-Starvation" in Derek Humphry's *Final Exit: The Practicalities of Self-Deliverance and Assisted Suicide for the Dying*. That chapter contains these sentences:

> Self-starvation has a distinct appeal for some. It is essentially an independent action, taking responsibility for your own death, involving no others in possibly illegal actions. It is demonstrating a desire to die at this point because of an unacceptable quality of life. (p. 62)

My friend Rebecca told me about a recent (2017) book by Phyllis Shacter, *Choosing to Die, a Personal Story: Elective*

Death by Voluntarily Stopping Eating and Drinking (VSED) in the Face of Degenerative Disease. I ordered a copy and read it right away. *Choosing to Die* is the story of the decision by Phyllis Shacter's husband Alan, who suffered from cancer and Alzheimer's disease, to stop eating and drinking. Alan knew from having taken care of his mother during her long and lingering years in the later stages of Alzheimer's that he wanted to find a way to die while he was still "competent" enough to make the decision about when and how to make it happen. He heard about VSED as a way to end his life easily, cheaply, and legally.

Alan and his wife talked with lawyers about whether patients can legally refuse treatments, procedures, medicines, food, and liquids that would keep them alive. They found out that it is perfectly legal, at least in the state of Washington.

And while doctors are not allowed to administer poisons or lethal injections—a practice known by various names like "assisted suicide," "euthanasia," and "murder"—they can prescribe drugs that will reduce or eliminate pain and anxiety in patients who voluntarily stop taking medicines, food, and liquids. Alan and Phyllis found out about what they needed to do to verify that Alan, despite his early affliction with Alzheimer's, was still mentally competent to make the decision about refusing food and water, and that he fully understood the consequences of that decision. They gathered the legal and medical documents they were advised to have on hand to head off possible interference from any family members, friends, neighbors, and government officials who might raise objections or try to accuse Phyllis of murder or spousal neglect.

They talked with doctors about what a VSED death was like, what help they would need during the actual process of starvation and dehydration, and what comfort measures would be needed to keep Alan pain-free. They selected a doctor who agreed to look in on Alan from time to time during his dying and to prescribe procedures, treatments, and medications, as needed. They lined up a hospice team that would provide twenty-four-hour surveillance and would do what they could to keep Alan comfortable and Phyllis calm.

Because little was publicly known about VSED at that time, Alan and Phyllis had little but their own curiosity and courage to guide them. After Alan's death on the tenth day after his VSED start-date, Phyllis Shacter decided to write *Choosing to Die* to help others learn about VSED, how to think about it, how to anticipate the problems that they might expect to face, and what the actual process of dying would be like from start-day to end-day. She recreated some of the conversations that she and her husband had in the months leading up to Alan's decision to die by VSED and his decision to pick a start-date. She describes the pre-death "funeral" they organized while Alan was still alive and able to enjoy the nice things his friends said about him.

Alan's decision to die by VSED was, of course, not easy for him. But it was hard for Phyllis, also. Already exhausted from years of dealing with her husband's Alzheimer's and his laryngeal cancer, she now found herself needing to deal with his dying. She writes about the frustration she felt when Alan picked a start-date for his VSED, then changed his mind and postponed—time and again. She talks about dealing with the lurking suspicions of others that she was, for selfish reasons, pushing her husband to take the VSED escape route: "I was in a deep state of despair and exhaustion," she writes. "One day I woke up and could not stop crying. As is true with many of us, I had a difficult time asking for help, but now I knew I had to. I was desperate" (pp. 114–15).

Phyllis describes the sort of help and support that she needed both during the pre-VSED decision-making and during the ten days of Alan's actual dying. She describes in the day-by-day process of Alan's dying; the changing color of his urine, the bedpans, the sponge baths, the diapers.

Although at least one doctor thought Alan showed signs of early Parkinson's, that diagnosis was not confirmed. Whatever

Alan's illnesses were, his wife's *Choosing to Die* can be helpful to those of us who do have late-stage Parkinson's and who want to rescue ourselves and our families from the years of helpless dependency that otherwise probably lie ahead.

The goal of VSED is to make life more tolerable for both the patient and the caregiver, but the actual experience of VSED death can be challenging to both. Apparently Alan had access to enough morphine and other drugs to be mostly free of the discomfort and anxiety often associated with dying. He had originally told the doctor that he wanted to be "sedated to comfort level right from the beginning of the process," but on the actual start day he told her "he wanted as little medication as possible because he wanted to be as conscious as possible throughout the process" (p. 72). Apparently he changed his mind because he realized that to be made fully "comfortable" would be to miss the last days of a life that he very much loved. He decided that to be conscious for a few days longer, even in pain, was better than to be essentially unconscious during those last days of dying. To be even partially conscious meant, however, that he suffered some of the pangs and discomfort of starvation and dehydration.

Alan's change of mind meant more suffering not only for Alan but also for his wife. Take, for example, this passage in Phyllis Shacter's book. She had given the members of Alan's hospice team explicit instructions about what to do if Alan requested food or water. They were on no account to give him either, but were instead to fetch her and let her deal with it. Alan did ask for water:

> This is what I said to him: "You said you want to die so you don't have to live into the later stages of Alzheimer's. I'm happy to give you water, but I want you to know that it will extend the amount of time it takes you to die. Would you like a glass of water, or would it be enough for me to spray mists of water into your mouth until you are

satisfied?" He understood my words and said the mists of water would be enough. I sprayed and sprayed, and he lapped up the water like a kitty. He seemed satisfied and did not ask for water again. (pp. 73–74)

It troubles me to think of Alan pathetically attempting to lap up mist "like a kitty," but it troubles me more to think of him suffering years of worse indignities.

Will I take the VSED trail? It is too early to say. With any luck at all, I will not live so long that I need to put myself and Anne through the stressful months of deciding to get on that trail and then the two or three weeks of being kept "comfortable" while I slowly dehydrate myself to death. Surely, the alternative—a long period of bed-bound dependency—is even worse. Recognizing that I may well wind up on the VSED trail, I have taken the precaution of leaving this letter with our family doctor:

> Dear Dr. _____:
> After several searching discussions with Anne, I have decided to let you know that when the time comes, I may want to end my life by what has come to be known as VSED (Voluntarily Stopping Eating and Drinking). When I select a starting date, I will stop taking the medicines that I have been taking for Parkinson's and pre-diabetes and I will refuse all foods and liquids. After that date I want no nourishment or hydration by mouth, tube, or intravenous injection.
> I ask your help in authorizing and instructing a hospice team to assist me, my wife, and my children by providing "comfort measures" so that my pain, discomfort, and anxiety are kept to a minimum during the one-to-three weeks of my dying. The hospice team will keep me clean and as comfortable as possible, but will be instructed to

give me no nourishment or liquid (in any form, including water sprays or ice chips).

I welcome the use of whatever drugs you want to give me to keep me comfortably sedated until the end. I have never experimented with any drugs more powerful than aspirin or Scotch (well, I tried marijuana twice, but to no effect), so feel free to give me a joyous send-off!

My dying can take place at home with a hospice team helping Anne, but I would probably prefer that after the first day I be moved to a nursing home or end-of-life facility where the trained and experienced staff have the equipment and the experience to deal with VSED clients. Beyond hospice staff and immediate family, I want no visitors. I will not be pretty to look at and will be about as fun to be with as a sun-parched octopus. Totally cut off from my Parkinson's meds, especially carbidopa/levodopa, I will be totally immobilized, and therefore unable even to shake hands with a guest. I would rather be remembered as I was when I was alive—active, vertical, and ugly—than as I will be in hospice—rigid, horizontal, and ugly. I do not want Anne or my children to have to clean me or my diapers or my clothes or my sheets or my bedsheets or my excretory messes.

Another advantage to my dying in a nursing facility is that it will facilitate the donation of my brain for Parkinson's research and the donation of the rest of my body to the University of Washington School of Medicine for instructional purposes.

I think I heard that Medicare will not pay for my VSED-oriented death unless I am brought to a hospital emergency ward in an ambulance. I am also aware that if I am taken from my home to an end-of-life care place, Medicare will pay for none of it and Anne will have to pay the entire cost of my hospital stay out-of-pocket. If that is the case, then I will want to do my VSED at home, with whatever hospice help you can authorize to help Anne care for me in my final days.

I ask that you do all you can for Anne. This VSED thing will be particularly difficult for her. She has lovingly fed me delicious and nutritious meals for most of sixty years. It will not be easy for her to witness my slow death by VSED. I do hope that you will ask from time to time how she is getting along.

You are no doubt wondering when my start-date will be. I do not know. I fall down four or five times a day. Surely in one of these falls I will break some bone or damage some vital organ. That will probably trigger VSED for me. Instead of asking you to fix me, Anne and I may ask you to consider that as my VSED start time.

Thank you!

Peter G. Beidler
(Date) _____

I guess I should leave a note like this when I actually begin VSED:

To whom it may concern:

After fifteen years of steadily growing weaker and less in control of my movements, I have decided that it is time for me to end my life by voluntarily stopping eating and drinking (VSED). With this note I declare my intention to deprive my body of all Parkinson's and diabetes medicines and to stop eating and drinking. I do so with the full knowledge that these actions will cause my death in a period of one to three weeks.

I ask that my family and hospice workers not try to give me food or drink. Doing so will only delay my dying. I ask that I be given palliative "comfort" medicines as prescribed by my medical team.

I thank my wife Anne and my four children, Paul, Kurt, Calloway, and Nora for making my living and my dying so joyful.

Sincerely,
Peter G. Beidler
(Date): _____

And while I am thinking of the letters I want to write, I want to thank my hospice team:

Hi. I'm Pete. When you meet me, I'm likely to be horizontal, unconscious, and pretty much out of it. Before I get that way, though, I want to seize an opportunity to thank you for helping Anne, my lovely wife of fifty-six years, to take care of what is left of me. I'd like to be able to thank you in person, but I guess that will not be possible. This letter, written not so long ago by the guy on the bed, will have to suffice. It is not a long letter. It can be summarized in two words: Thank you.

I thank you for your willingness to help Anne and our children deal with the body of a man who is dying. I would have enjoyed getting to know you under friendlier and more sociable circumstances. I would have asked about where you were born and raised, whether you have siblings or children, how you first became interested in hospice service.

By the time you are summoned to my bedside, however, I will have begun the serious business of dying. I will probably have taken a bad fall, or been infected with pneumonia, or have had, as both my parents did, a stroke. I apologize for the unpleasantness of the work that lies ahead for you as a member of my hospice team.

I think of hospice workers as end-of-life midwives. Like birthing midwives, or doulas, you deal with the sometimes painful, usually messy, transitions between being and not-being, and between life and death. You deal with the excretions and odors and stains and filth of bodies in transition.

I wish you could have known me before I became so horizontal. It is probably difficult for you to imagine that this inert and bedfast body once belonged to a funny, ambitious, lively, engaged person. I do wish I could be more entertaining. You deserve more fun in your life than I can give you now.

I want you to know that I have been incredibly lucky. I had almost perfect health for seventy-five years, before my Parkinson's made me stumble and fall so often. I had a perfect wife, four perfect children, and nine perfect grandchildren. I had a wonderful job as a teacher. I got to live in wonderful places like Seattle. I had wonderful friends. And I got to be cared for in my closeout days by wonderful people like you.

Thank you!
Peter G. Beidler
(Date):_____

19. The ABCs of Self-Deliverance

IN THE PREVIOUS SEVERAL CHAPTERS I tried to show that we people with Parkinson's are able to exert some control over *how* and *where* we die. In this chapter I take up the more difficult question of taking control of *when* we die. On the one hand, we should be grateful that the disease progresses so slowly, because its slow pace gives us a relatively long period of pretty good health in which to continue our professions, work our way through our bucket lists, write that novel we always wanted to write, visit old friends and relatives, make peace with our enemies, get our financial affairs in order, and so on. On the other hand, the slow progress of the disease means that when the going gets rough, as it almost invariably does, it stays rough for a long time.

I have two older sisters. Jo, three years older, lived a half-hour's drive from my home in eastern Pennsylvania. I saw her often. Sue, two years older, married an Englishman and emigrated with him to Australia, where she worked over the years as a palliative care nurse. She administered the medical needs for hundreds of old and dying women at a nursing home for elderly women near Sydney. Every five years or so, Sue flew back to the U.S. to visit. On one of those visits I picked her up at the Philadelphia airport. As we drove north to our house, I told her about Jo's health. When I mentioned that Jo had just been diagnosed with Parkinson's, Sue wept.

"Oh no," she said. "Anything but *that*. Parkinson's takes forever. Is she in a nursing home?"

"Goodness, no. She's fine. You'll see. She's coming down for dinner with us tonight. She wants to ask you what you know about Parkinson's."

"She must be in the early stages, then. I never see them until much later. Thanks for telling me. She will not want to hear what I have to say about Parkinson's, so I'll shut up about it. It's just about the last disease that any nurse would want to have."

"Jo told me it's not so bad," I said. "She has pills she takes that help a lot. She realizes that eventually her Parkinson's will get kind of bad, but her doctor said he is not even sure that's what it is. He told her they would keep an eye on it. If it is Parkinson's, he told her, the prognosis for a cure is very good."

"Good," Sue replied. "I'll stay out of it. I really don't know much about the early stages, and there is no reason that Jo needs to hear what I could say about the later stages."

"You can tell me," I said. "I don't have Parkinson's." At the time, l thought that was true. I didn't get diagnosed until several years later.

It was Sue's nature to be blunt and talkative. "I've taken care of lots of old ladies with Parkinson's," she said. "By the time I see them in the nursing home, they are pretty far along—so far along that they can no longer manage on their own. They have to be taken care of by family members at home. When I see them, they often cannot get out of bed without assistance, cannot dress themselves, feed themselves, get to the toilet, wipe or bathe themselves. Some cannot swallow efficiently, so we have to give them only very soft food, very wet soups, or regular food that we puree for them into a liquid goo. For some, we finally have to resort to feeding them through a feeding tube that bypasses the alimentary canal altogether. Some of the ladies seem to be mentally sharp, as near as I can tell. But how can I tell? Most of them cannot talk clearly enough that I can understand them. There is little we can do for them except keep them alive. We keep track of their meds, feed them, clean them, dress them, and prop them up so they can watch stupid programs on the telly. They rarely get visitors because there is little reward for the visitor. We have a couple of loyal husbands who come in every day, but they spend more time talking with us nurses than with their wives. We at least smile and answer their questions. We always try to spiff up the lucky wives of such men. You know, comb their hair, pinch a little color into their cheeks, dab some makeup here and there, pick out a nice blouse for them to wear. Poor Jo. I wonder how much of this she knows."

"Probably not much." I said. "Is it always so grim?"

"Not if they die of something before we get them. But by the time we get them in the nursing home, that's pretty much the way it seems to go. Of course, there are lots of variations. But I will tell you this: I never saw one of the Parkinson's ladies get better and walk out of the place. Once they come to us, they die with us."

"So, is that the way Jo will end up—immobilized in a nursing home, waiting to die?"

"Maybe. Everyone's story is different."

"That sounds like a miserable way to die."

"You would hate it, Pete, just hate it. You always have to be DOING something. These Parkinson's ladies can't DO much of anything."

"Jo still does plenty, but she does it more slowly. Oh well, I guess we all have to die of something, don't we? It could be worse. She could have a brain tumor or cancer or a massive heart attack."

"I'd take any one of those over Parkinson's."

"Really? Even cancer? Cancer can be painful."

"Absolutely. Cancer can be painful and fatal and even

sometimes curable. But at least it makes up its mind. Parkinson's just drags on and on, nibbling away at your ability to move, to take care of yourself. Cancer leaves you a corpse, but a dead corpse. For too many years Parkinson's leaves you a living corpse, a kind of zombie. With cancer, you know you're dead. With Parkinson's, you might as well be dead, but you're not. Parkinson's just goes on and on, quietly robbing you of one skill after another. It never gets better."

It is interesting how life works out. A year later, Sue was diagnosed with stage three lung cancer. As a young woman, she smoked cigarettes to keep her weight down. After years of treating smokers who often died of lung cancer, Sue gave up smoking.

For the next twenty-five years, Sue did not smoke. But the damage was done, and a year after that visit to Jo and me in Pennsylvania, Jo and I and our little sister Fran flew to Sydney, Australia, to say goodbye to Sue. It was a sad trip, of course, but a good one. Jo did fine despite her Parkinson's. I was happy for Sue that she got her wish to die of something quick.

Two years after that, when Jo was still doing pretty well with her Parkinson's, I was given my own diagnosis. Before I share my own thoughts about a long, slow death by Parkinson's, I want to finish up my sister Jo's story.

As Sue had predicted, things did get worse and then still worse as Jo's disease progressed. It got so she rarely left her wheelchair. She lost weight, but not because she tried to. No, she lost weight because she ate so much more slowly than the others. They started to clear the table when she was still chewing and swallowing the second bite. She did not want to hold up the others, so she pretended she was full.

This past fall (2018), after Jo had lived with the disease for more than fifteen years, things started getting pretty rough. By then in her early eighties, Jo still lived in their rural home with Bjarne, her husband of more than sixty years, but she stumbled and fell often, and could scarcely feed or take care of herself.

At eighty-nine, Bjarne was in better health than Jo, but their daughters worried that caring for Jo might seriously damage his health. They decided it was time for Jo to go into Gracedale, a nearby county nursing home. After two months there, in the early spring of 2019, Jo died.

Influencing when we die. I assume that my mother, my sister Sue, and my sister Jo all had on file witnessed statements about whether they wanted to be allowed to die a natural death or preferred to be kept alive by the use of artificial electronic or mechanical equipment. In signing those advance directives, they were attempting to take charge, in a small way, of their own death narratives. They did not want to leave entirely to chance or to the judgment of others decisions about when they might die. They wanted to inform their medical teams and members of their families about their preferences.

One of the most distressing features of Parkinson's is that it involves a slow, steady, expensive decline into unproductive and dependent helplessness, and sometimes into dementia. Some of us with the disease think that we may want to do more than tell our families to hold the feeding tubes and the breathing machines. We think we may someday want to consider some form of self-deliverance, maybe the way called VSED. But how do we know when it is time to take such action?

To help me figure out when it is time to begin my voluntary self-deliverance, I worked up a series of questions. My honest answers might give me clues about when to take active steps to avoid that long, expensive, unproductive, and unfun pre-death period we so dread. These questions may prove helpful to others who seek to exercise some control over how long they want to keep swimming in the murky twilight waters of River Parkinson. Probably we can never know for sure, but my answers should help me decide whether the time for my exit is drawing near. So far my own answers tell me, "Drawing near, yes, Pete, but not quite yet."

But this chapter is about you, not me. If you are wondering

whether it is time for you to consider self-deliverance, you might read through these twenty-six questions. There is no scoring except your own feelings. If most of the questions seem troubling to you, you are perhaps wondering how much longer you want to insist on staying alive. If your honest answers to some of the questions involve your telling yourself little fibs, maybe you should ask yourself why. Perhaps answering these smaller questions will help you to unpack your thinking about the larger one.

    a. Which do I anticipate with more eagerness, the coming of morning when I need to get up and do something or the coming of night when I can lie down and rest?

    b. Do I want my family and friends to remember me as I am now or as I will perhaps be, say, two years from now?

    c. Is there some unfinished work I want to complete before I sign out?

    d. Am I still well enough, and motivated enough, to finish that work?

    e. Does the work I want to do need doing?

    f. Who will benefit from my doing it, and how?

    g. Would I want the job of taking care of me for the next two years?

    h. If I manage to stay alive for two more years, at whose expense will it be?

    i. To what extent am I now dependent on others for my daily care—feeding, bathing, dressing, getting around, reading, exercising?

    j. How rapid is my Parkinson's decline?

    k. Do I feel myself descending into dementia?

    l. If there is evidence that I am becoming demented, have I let the key decision-makers in my life know, in writing, how vigorously I do not want to be kept alive as my dementia worsens?

m. What am I still capable of doing that will help other people? Am I still doing it?

n. Is my duel with death winnable?

o. In my duel with death, what constitutes a victory?

p. Would I be better off gracefully conceding and so avoiding the unenviable pummeling that lies ahead?

q. Do I want to live longer for my own benefit or for the benefit of someone else?

r. If the former, how precisely will I benefit from more alive-time? If the latter, how precisely will that person benefit from my living a little longer?

s. If I want to do what is best for the people I love most—my care partner and my children—what path will I take?

t. If I opt to live longer, from whose pockets will the money come that will pay for private-duty nursing care in my home or for professional care in a nursing home? From whose pockets will come my wheelchair, my wheelchair ramp, my wheelchair-accessible van?

u. If I am experiencing pain, is there a non-addictive way to get relief from the pain?

v. If I won a $10 million lottery tomorrow, how would I spend the money?

w. If I could take a two-week journey to anywhere in the world, where would I go—or would I stay home?

x. It has been said that we need three things to be happy: something to do, someone to love, and hope for a better life. Do I have all three? Is it enough to have only two of them? Only one?

y. If everyone who had my disease and my symptoms were to choose as I am about to choose, would that be a good thing?

z. Is my decision about self-deliverance a choice between life and death, or is it really a choice between death and death: a sooner, cheaper, cleaner death on my own terms or a later, more expensive, and messier death on someone else's terms?

We have some important choices to consider, don't we? They are scary choices, but they are *our* choices—our *joyous* choices. We cannot count on the solace of a cure for our Parkinson's. We cannot count on the solace of an escape from eventual death. But perhaps we can, by giving serious thought to questions like these, know that we have taken important steps toward influencing the time, the circumstances, and the spirit of our dying.

In the next chapter, I indicate the direction my choices are now tending toward. You will make different choices—but that is what choice is all about, isn't it? The point is that we are not trapped in a dark, one-way-only tunnel. We have the solace of choice.

Take charge, boss!

20. The Way Ahead

[Several years ago, in the spring of 2015, I sent an early draft of the following letter to my wife and my four children. In the spring of 2019, I updated it to reflect my more recent thinking and my reading of a few books not available in 2015. I include this revised letter because it might give you some ideas for your own letter expressing your own thoughts and desires about what lies ahead. Your letter, of course, will be different from mine because it will be yours.*]*

DEAR ANNE, PAUL, KURT, CALLOWAY, AND Nora:
As you know, I have had a relatively easy journey so far with my Parkinson's. I pretty much did what I wanted to do, went where I wanted to go, ate what I wanted to eat, built what I wanted to build, wrote what I wanted to write. But the good days are drawing to a close. I take more and more carbidopa/ levodopa pills, but they do almost no good now. I have long since given up driving, and sometimes even getting into or out of the passenger side of a car is a challenge. I have difficulty speaking now, and my auditors can rarely understand me. I can scarcely walk without a walker, and even when I try to walk with a walker, I often cannot move my feet. I fall down, on

average, three or four times a day. It is getting more and more difficult for me to get up from these falls. One of these times I will not be able to get up. I seem to have tough old bones, since none have broken in any of my falls, but one of these days my luck will run out. I still feed myself (though I spill a lot). I still bathe myself (though the soap has a way of slipping out of my hands). I still keep track of my own meds (though Anne occasionally finds a little yellow pill on the floor). I still change the delicate batteries on my hearing aids (but the tiny wax guards are too small for my quivering hands).

I have a strong sense that I need to make some decisions about how I want to approach the difficult times ahead. I am painfully aware, of course, that my decisions have profound implications for the rest of my family—particularly for Anne.

In *A Parkinson's Life and a Caregiver's Roadmap* (2018), Jolyon Hallows describes in ominous detail the twenty-year saga of his experience as the caregiver of his wife Sandra, who had suffered for years with Parkinson's. The book contains lessons for all of us, but I want to quote a particularly sad passage near the end:

> Just after New Year's, she came down with the flu and spent three weeks in hospital. For most of it, she was minimally responsive and on a nasal feeding tube. One of her doctors told me that if she didn't start swallowing, they would have to insert a feeding tube into her abdomen—and what kind of quality of life would that give her? That was a blunt, realistic question. The doctor's advice was to start end-of-life planning. That was the toughest day I had faced. A few times during our marriage, I had broached the subject of death with Sandra. Neither of us would live forever and I wanted to know her preferences. But every time I raised it, she either ignored me or changed the topic. It was not something she was willing to discuss. So now, the decision was solely mine

and I had to face the question: What will I do? (p. 181)

I do not want to ignore the topic of death or change the subject, as Sandra Hallows did. It seems that the very least I can do for you five is to state, in writing, as clearly as I can, why my end-of-life preference is for brevity rather than longevity.

First, however, let me state what I hope is obvious: that I consider myself to have been blessed by the best wife and children any man could dream of. If I have, despite my errors and shortcomings, been a generally acceptable husband and father, it is because you five have made it easy, fun, and rewarding. I am grateful to you all, but to beautiful Anne first and forever, for making my long life so pleasant and for filling the houses we have occupied—in Richmond (Indiana), Bethlehem and Easton (Pennsylvania), Tucson and Polacca (Arizona), Waco (Texas), Canterbury (England), Chengdu (China), and Seattle (Washington)—with such happiness.

You all know that Parkinson's is a progressive, incurable neurodegenerative disease. Medications (especially carbidopa/levodopa) and surgery (especially deep brain stimulation or DBS) can help mask some of the symptoms for some patients for a while, but they do not stop or necessarily even slow down the disease itself.

I have been told that, because of my age and my particular Parkinson's symptoms, I am not a "candidate" for deep brain stimulation. Other therapies, like nutritional supplements and exercise, can help, but Parkinson's inevitably wins in the end. With my meds, with Anne's nutritional expertise, and with exercise, I have been fortunate to have had a relatively trouble-free first decade with the disease. But the FOG (freezing of gait) that sometimes comes as the disease advances is now growing increasingly troublesome, causing me to stumble often and fall down a lot. Falls are dangerous. I could of course protect myself from falling by yielding to the wheelchair and the bed, but I am sure you understand why I am reluctant to yield. For an old man approaching eighty, life in a wheelchair is not life. A life confined to a bed is not life. Such a "life," for me, would be worse than death.

What I do not want for me. As I approach the finish line, I do not want the long period of dying that Parkinson's seems to send to most of us with this disease. That is, I do not want an extensive, expensive, exhausting, and funless decline in which I slowly, reluctantly, but relentlessly lose the ability to move, act, think, read, build, play, write, and speak. In the natural course of events, what probably lies ahead for me as a man with advanced Parkinson's is an extended period of invalidism. How far ahead that will be, of course, and how long it will last, no one can say. I do not want any part of it. I have always defined myself primarily by doing—by working, by walking, by building houses, bookshelves, and toys, by playing games, by putting together picture puzzles, by thinking, by writing, by publishing, by learning, by traveling, by reading, by helping others with little projects. The prospect of an extended period of what I might call nondoing or undoing is abhorrent to me.

What I want for me. I am not afraid of being dead, but I am a little afraid of dying—that is, of the process of getting dead. Being dead will be calm, peaceful, quiet. Dying a Parkinson's death will probably be variously unpleasant: painful, expensive, messy, undignified, drawn-out, and humiliating. I want to find a way to cheat the end stages of Parkinson's—the wheelchair-ridden and bedridden stages that are the eventual endings for most people with the disease. I am not sure how I will do that, but I hope you will let me or help me do it my way. If I can't get myself out of bed, dress myself, or get around, even with my cane, my walker, my rollator (wheeled walker), or my wheeled knee-walker, then, hey, okay, the game is over. Bed baths, bedside commodes, diapers, and bed sores—thanks, but no thanks. I'll pass. Especially obnoxious to me is the prospect of feeding tubes pumping baby-food-like goo into my stomach, or metering medicines into my intestine.

Almost as bad as tube feeding is the prospect of being spoon-fed by others when I can no longer feed myself. Please, no assistive feeding. If Pete can't or won't pick up, peel, chew, and swallow a banana, then no banana for Pete. Okay? If Pete can't or won't lift the pills and glass, then no water for Pete. And if Pete can't breathe, don't hook me up to a bicycle pump wheezing air into my lungs. Bike tires need that kind of air. I don't.

Death with dignity. Death is inevitable. The kind of senselessly prolonged dying that Parkinson's provides is evitable. Fortunately, I live in a state that has death with dignity laws in place. Unfortunately, these laws do not much help people with Parkinson's. As I understand it, the laws provide that if two doctors will certify that they believe a patient has less than six months to live, then that patient can get permission to end his or her life by swallowing a handful of pills or a flask of liquid medicine prescribed by one of the doctors.

There are several catches built into the death with dignity laws. The first is the difficulty of predicting how soon a Parkinson's patient will die "naturally." Doctors are understandably reluctant to risk malpractice suits by offering to predict the unpredictable. A second problem is that the law stipulates that patients must be able to lift the pills and the glass of liquid to their own lips, unassisted, and swallow them. In the last six months of their lives, some Parkinson's patients have lost the muscle control to lift the pills and the glass of water, or they have lost the ability to swallow the pills without choking. Death with dignity laws were not written with Parkinson's patients in mind.

On the contrary, the death with dignity laws virtually guarantee that, unless we have a blessed accident, kill ourselves in some sort of violent way (bullet, drowning, plastic bag, automobile exhaust, noose, and so on), or get serious about VSED, we will suffer a slow, laborious, disheartening death without dignity.

No, VSED does not stand for Vigorous Sex Every Day. As you know, I have been thinking recently about the various advantages of voluntarily stopping eating and drinking: it is legal; it has been used with some success by others; doctors are less reluctant to prescribe morphine than a more lethal medicine; hospice teams have had some experience with it; it gives families time to get used to the idea of death; and, most important, it gives late-stage Parkinson's patients a way to control the timing and the manner of our dying.

I do not fear too soon a death so much as I fear too long a life. I do not dread dying so much as I dread not dying— living past the time when I am capable of learning new things, enjoying old memories, building new things, enjoying a stupid old joke, talking with people I love or like, playing pool, poker, Hearts, Scrabble, Five-hundred, Casino, or Peanuts, writing letters like this. Life without all that would for me be worse than death. Spare me such a death-life. Help me get on to the real thing. Please?

What I do not want for you. Typically, the long, slow dying of a person with Parkinson's depletes the energies, patience, health, and financial and emotional resources of the people he or she would most like to spare such depletion. I have seen that depletion close at hand: Aunt Bea, Gorman, and Jo, to mention only family members; Vic Hays, Lou Cavazel, Gordon Hastings, Mary Larsen, Ralph Moldauer, and other friends I have made in the Parkinson's community here in Seattle. I have seen the toll Parkinson's takes on the care partners—the survivors, the families. I have seen the strain, the frustration, the waste, the guilt, the deprivation, the depletion, the anger. I want none of those for any of you.

One of Anne's biggest joys has always been her close association with our children and grandchildren. I do not want my prolonged dying to rob her of that joy by making her spend most of the rest of her old age taking care of an invalid old man. Nor do I want paid strangers to take care of me—except perhaps in the closing couple of weeks of VSED. While I am happy to provide employment to the unfortunate people who do such work for a living, and while I am happy to have them relieve Anne of some of the burden of caring for me, these paid helpers can do me little good. They merely prolong the miserable ending to a wonderful life.

A wonderful life? Sure. Mine truly has been a wonderful life, a life of love, learning, adventure, discovery, travel, friends, colleagues, students, writing, walking, games, reading, joking, raising amazing children, building functional and beautiful things of wood and stone. I would gladly have many more years of all that. The prospect of many more years without any of that, however, horrifies me. From the start I had good opportunities in education, travel, employment, homes to live in. I had a lovable, loving, and lovely wife and four stunning children. I have nine amazing grandchildren. I do not want your memories of that wonderful life to be crowded out by more recent memories of a less-than-wonderful closing period of pain, of assorted indignities, of pills, of walkers, of wheelchairs, of bedpans, of bed sores, of pointless expenses.

I have not taken out a long-term-care insurance policy in part because I did not want to pay the enormous premiums, but mostly because I do not want to be cared for in a long-term kind of way. If I were the kind of man who wanted to buy insurance, I would want it to be the kind of insurance that assured a shorter life. I do not want some faceless insurance company (or Medicare or Medicaid fund) to keep me alive. I draw a distinction between needing and wanting. I may well need long-term care if I am to stay alive, but I do not want it.

What I want for you. I want you all to be free of the need to take care of me. Parkinson's has at best a questionable right to trouble my closing years. It has no right whatever to trouble yours. I confess that part of my reluctance to seek a prolonged or extended life is financial. Anne and I have worked hard, invested cautiously, and spent frugally. I do not want the money we have managed to save to go for futile medical care in my last years. That is absolutely not what the working, investing, and frugal spending were for. That money is earmarked not to keep me alive past the time when I should have died; it is for you, my amazing Anne and then for you, our amazing children.

I retired from teaching when I was at or near the top of my game. I wanted to leave before people started wondering why I was still around. I'd like to retire from living before it is painfully obvious that there is no longer any point in my being around.

Marcus and Marty. The deaths of our two neighbors in the little village of Coffeetown, Pennsylvania, influenced my thinking about how I want to die. You all remember Marcus Nicholas. He was in his early seventies when I asked him one sunny June morning if he would help me saw a limb off a tree. He said "Sure" and brought his chainsaw over. I set a ladder up against the tree. Marcus climbed the ladder and started the chainsaw. It took only a moment to cut through the limb. As the limb hit the ground, however, it took a cruel bounce. The sawed end of the limb jumped back and hit the base of the ladder and knocked it away from the tree. Marcus fell to the ground, hitting his head against a rock. I cradled him in my arms until the ambulance came. Three hours later he was declared dead by a doctor at the Easton Hospital emergency ward.

None of us knew Marcus's next-door neighbor, Marty Kester, as well as we knew Marcus. Marty had multiple sclerosis. The disease slowly robbed him over the years of his ability to work, to climb stairs, to walk, to eat, to swallow, to talk. My last memory of Marty is of him sitting on his front porch in his wheelchair, chain-smoking cigarettes and watching the cars go by. Then he could no longer even get out to the porch. He finally died about three years after that. I heard that during most of his last three years, his wife Edna fed him with a funnel hooked up to a feeding tube, the other end of which was surgically inserted into his stomach. Marty had more years, but Marcus had more life.

Margaret and Mariemma. My mother, Margaret Beidler and Anne's mother, Mariemma Gilbert, both died not long after they had massive strokes. They never quite came to after their strokes, and we children all had to make decisions about how vigorously we should try to keep them alive. In both cases, guided by their own pre-death directives, we helped to ease them over the great divide by withholding tube-nourishment and force-feeding. I ask, when my time comes, to be allowed to die as naturally and as quickly as possible. No artificial respiration. No feeding tubes, no shoving food into my mouth, no intravenous nourishment or hydration. If I get pneumonia, let me die from it rather than pumping me full of antibiotics or oxygen in an effort to rescue me from it. There is a reason they call pneumonia an old man's friend. Let's allow it to be friendly. If I have a stroke, if I have a heart attack, if I fall and hurt myself pretty badly, if I get cancer, if I am in an automobile accident, if my pre-diabetic condition takes a sudden turn south .... Well, you get the idea. Remember, the thought of being dead is far more appealing to me than the thought of being uselessly alive.

Some doctors, nurses, and emergency medical technicians will want to resuscitate me so that I can live longer. It is what they are trained to do, what they are paid to do, what they think the law requires them to do, and what they think I would of course want them to do. They will want to bring me back from the gate and keep me alive. Only you, armed with this statement, my advance directive, and my POLST forms (see below), can stop them.

Stop them.

POLST form. The Washington State Medical Association provides a bright green 8.5-by-11-inch form which is to be used to guide the responses of emergency medical technicians (EMTs) and hospital staff. The idea is that they will find the form displayed in a prominent place in my house or, if I am in an automobile accident, in my car. I usually carry a copy of the form in my wallet. "POLST" stands for Physician Orders for Life-Sustaining Treatment. It is curiously named. For one thing, the form expresses not the physician's orders but the patient's. We decide which boxes to check. The physician does not issue the orders, but merely witnesses our orders. The name is curious also because the purpose of the document is to stipulate what kind of life-sustaining treatments *not* to give. The bright green POLST form has two sides. Specifically, on my POLST form I request that the EMT medical people, if they find no pulse, allow a natural death and that they not transfer me to a hospital. More to the point for people with Parkinson's, I ask for no feeding tubes, no transfusion of medical products, no dialysis. To use a sports analogy, it means that I want no overtime, no extra innings. My family doctor at the Ballard branch of the Swedish Medical Center discussed the form with me in the presence of Anne. The doctor's signature certifies that I signed the form voluntarily and with full knowledge of the implications of what I was doing.

My brain and my body. I have made plans and signed documents to donate what is left after I shuffle off this mortal coil for scientific research and educational purposes. My brain goes to the University of Washington's Pacific Northwest Udall Center (PANUC) for research into the causes and courses of Parkinson's disease. It is vital that this call be made almost immediately after death. One of the advantages of VSED is that the people watching over my final days will be able to predict with a fair degree of accuracy how much longer it will be before I die. I suggest that someone call the PANUC folks when death is imminent to alert them to the situation and to receive instructions about picking up my body.

The rest of me goes toward the education of medical students at the University of Washington Medical Center. I've spent most of my life as a teacher, and it pleases me to know that I can go on teaching after I die.

I guess that says it all. I would add only that I had thought writing this letter would be depressing. It has not been. On the contrary, writing it leaves me feeling more delighted than depressed. It feels good to let you know how I feel about the issues we six will face together in the near or distant future.

How unusual is it for me to welcome and embrace death as a friend rather than fight or run from it as an enemy? To show that more and more men and women are starting to question the death-as-enemy model, I refer you to a recent video and offer brief quotations from four recent books about death. The video was produced in the Seattle area by Trudy Brown. Called *Speaking of Dying*, it deals openly and compassionately with many of the issues that confront dying patients and their families. The first of the recent books about death and dying is Dr. Atul Gawande's *Being Mortal* (2014). Dr. Gawande is critical of medical schools for not preparing doctors to deal more realistically with death. He is critical of himself for thinking of his patients as bodies rather than fellow human beings. And he is critical of society for encouraging people to buy into the idea that death is an obstacle to be overcome rather than a natural and universal condition to be embraced:

> You don't have to spend much time with the elderly or those with terminal illness to see how often medicine fails the people it is supposed to help. The waning days of our lives are given over to treatments that addle our brains and sap our bodies for a sliver's chance of benefit. They are spent in institutions—nursing homes and intensive care units—where regimented, anonymous routines cut us off from all the things that matter to us in life. (p. 9)

A second book about death and dying is sociologist and theologian Stephen Jenkinson's *Die Wise* (2015). Jenkinson is particularly concerned in the book about people who think that death is something to be resisted, delayed, fought, and cured.

Dying is a natural thing, and left to its natural self each living thing knows how to die. The body has the genius of a natural thing, and it knows how to obey the accumulation of time, wear and tear, disease and symptoms. It knows how to stop. But med-tech, not in any sense a natural thing, knows how to subvert the way disease and symptoms have of keeping and marking time, and in doing so it subverts the body's knowledge of how to stop. (p. 51)

A third book is Paul Kalanithi's *When Breath Becomes Air* (2016). Dr. Kalanithi was a neurosurgeon who usually tried to rescue his patients from death, but sometimes had to recognize—and help families recognize—that death was actually preferable to a post-surgical "life." The "they" in the quotation below are members of the family of a patient who has been severely brain-damaged by an accident or a disease. The "I" is Dr. Kalanithi, the surgeon:

In these moments, I acted not, as I most often did, as death's enemy; but as its ambassador. I had to help those families understand that the person they knew—the full, vital, independent human—now lived only in the past and that I needed their input to understand what sort of future he or she would want: an easy death or to be strung between bags of fluid going in, others coming out. (pp. 87 –88)

A fourth recent book about death and dying is Dr. Jessica Nutik Zitter's *Extreme Measures* (2018). Dr. Zitter talks about her many years of experience in dealing with the very sick and often dying patients in the "trenches" of her dehumanizing intensive care unit (ICU). She describes her growing dissatisfaction with the hospital culture that denies the individual humanity of the patients sent to her ICU. She describes her growing resistance to assuming that they all *want* to live as long as possible no matter what the cost. She asks that doctors make the effort to find out what their patients want in the way of medical care in their closing weeks. She asks that patients think about what sort of death they want, share their thoughts with their doctors and family members, and have on file a written advance directive that can help determine the manner, the duration, the cost, and the level of comfort of their dying:

> I came to see that in our zeal to save life, we often worsened death. (p. 47)

> Over 50 percent of Americans die in pain. Seventy percent die in institutions. And 30 percent of families lose most of their life savings while caring for a dying loved one. (p. 50)

Do I want to spend $5,000 a day uselessly prolonging my life in an intensive care unit? Do I want to end my days with a breathing machine pumping air into my lungs through a surgical incision in my neck? Do I want to die with large catheters stuck into every possible orifice?

You know how I would answer those questions. I love you all!

Peter G. Beidler

21. Where's Grandpa?

DEAR PETER, WILLOW, LUCAS, MERLIN, MARCUS, Elowyn, Hugo, Annie, and Elizabeth:

Perhaps you're wondering where I am now. You all knew, of course, that the end was coming. You all saw me lurch and stumble these last couple of years. You saw me freeze stupidly when I tried to walk through a doorway or get on or off an elevator or escalator.

You saw me stop unaccountably when I tried to cross a street, and you hoped that the cars and busses would see me and stop before mowing me down.

You saw me dribble my drool and slop my soup when I tried to eat.

You heard my voice get weaker and my words get more garbled and stuttery when I tried to talk. You noticed as time went on that I spoke less and less. You'll recall that I never had a whole lot to say, anyhow, but you noticed that I was more apt to use hand signals than words. Instead of asking for a glass of water so I could take some little yellow pills, I handed you my empty glass and mimicked with my right hand a tipping pitcher.

Instead of saying "It's your turn to deal," I pointed to the deck of cards and then to you.

And you perhaps noticed that I never answered the phone anymore. Nobody could really understand me on the phone anymore. People learned to call Anne, instead, or to text me or email me. Giving up talking was difficult. Speech is one of the abilities that makes us human. To lose that ability makes me feel like a dog. I can wag my tail and say "Arf" but that is not the same as talking, now, is it? "Bow-wow?"

You heard the little buzzer in my pocket go off to remind me every two hours to take another fistful of pills. You saw me get on the senior citizens Access bus that came twice a week to take me to my Yoga for People with Parkinson's class or to the gym where I took part in an exercise program known as Rock Steady Boxing. You could see that I was anything but steady as a rock.

You noticed my world grow smaller as I gave up driving, then gave away my beloved Suburban, then gave up walking. Giving up walking was especially hard. I loved walking. When we first moved to Seattle, I walked miles and miles every day: to the gym, to the bus stops, to the post office. Perhaps you sensed how frustrating it was for me to realize I could no longer even walk safely around the block.

You knew the end was coming for me, but my death may leave you wondering where I went and where I am now. You probably know about the physical part of me—the part I have donated "to science." I have signed papers donating my brain— after my death, of course!—for research on Parkinson's disease. And as for the rest of my physical body, from the nose to the toes, I have donated it to the University of Washington School of Medicine to help medical students learn about basic human anatomy. But the rest of me, the more important part of me? Where is that? I wish I could answer that question, but of course I cannot.

I don't really buy into the concepts of heaven and hell, but they are not relevant to me anyhow. If there is a heaven, I've not been angelic enough to gain admittance, and if there is a hell, I've not been diabolical enough to get sent there. So where am I? I guess the best I can do is tell you that I am now where I was before I was born. Where do babies come from? Oh, I know, you understand about basic biology, about sexual intercourse and eggs and sperms and gestation and wombs and labor and birth and suddenly!—a baby. But that is all just physical stuff. The question here is, where that baby was before sexual intercourse brought the egg and the wiggly sperm together? Where was that baby before she or he was conceived, before there was a physical Baby Grandpa? Where that baby was then is kind of where I am now.

How is that for a non-answer?

There is an expression that may help here: "That happened before you were born, Sonny, back when you were nothing more than a gleam in your old man's eye." That is kind of like what I am now. When I died, the gleam went out of my eye. But there is still a gleam in the eye of my children and my surviving friends. You'll recognize me in that gleam of pride when you have a birthday or when you graduate with some degree or when you accomplish something special. I'll be in that gleam, still grinning like a stupid idiot. You'll see a gleam in your parents' eyes as they grin like idiots when you do something spectacular like ace a test, play a solo in the jazz band, throw the winning frisbee in the final game of the Ultimate season, get your SAT scores back, build a jewelry box in your workshop, bake your mother a birthday cake, whatever. If you stop to think about it, you'll know that I am part of that gleam.

That is one way to answer where I am now. Another way is to say that I am in what I have left behind: in my stunning wife (the gracious grandmother who has helped more emphatically than I to raise you); in my stunning children (your stunning parents); in what I have built (mills, houses, porches, bookshelves, carvings, toys, boats, coffee tables). And you will see me in what I have written. Most of what I have written will be of no interest to you. But there are some bits that may have meaning for you—like a few of the essays in my little book, *Risk Teaching* (my "Educational Autobiography," "Why I Teach," "What's Your Horse," and even "Pat the Cat"). I have also been writing down some of my memories of my early life. These can be found in a little book called *Ambles*, now in private production. If you ever get curious about what my own youth was like, perhaps you can get your mom or dad to make you a copy.

There are a few other things I would like to say to you now, in writing. I've lived a pretty long time and have learned a few things about life and love and marriage and what is important, and how to get along in the world. Some of these may be of interest to you as you embark on new phases of your own lives. I hope I come off sounding wise, not preachy, but I will almost certainly fail to achieve that hope. Still, preachy or not, here I come.

You have two huge decisions ahead of you. One is the kind of work you will do.

What kind of work to do. Try lots of jobs along the way: wait tables, drive taxis, mow lawns, babysit, carry lumber, fix lawn mowers, wash cars, mix concrete, milk cows, flip hamburgers. You might be surprised at how much fun menial work can be and how much fun you can have with your fellow workers. Save most of your money and treasure your experiences and friends. But keep your eye on your main goal: to find out in the process what you most like to do. As you select your life's work, keep in mind that what you really want is to find a way to have someone pay you to do what you would do for the pure fun of it. On the other hand, if what you really enjoy is writing poetry or planting marigolds in south-facing window boxes, those activities will probably not earn you a living wage. As you pursue your education and seek employment, keep an eye out for what people are willing to pay you for. There are lots of jobs worth doing that will let you write poetry or plant marigolds in your spare time. Prepare yourself for such jobs.

Who to marry. The other big decision is who to marry. Falling in love is an emotional thing; go with your heart. Getting married is more an intellectual thing: go with your brain. Before you wed, ask yourself the tough questions: will he be a steady husband? Will she be a loving mother? Is he careful with money? Will she be a steady wife? Will he be a loving father? Is she careful with money? Can he cook? Can she take the garbage out? Can one of you fix a car? Can one of you do the taxes? Fall in love early and often. Try to get married only once. Date a few Jaguars, some MGs, a couple of Corvettes, but marry a Honda Accord. It is less exotic, but requires less maintenance, is more versatile, and takes the potholes better. It is easy as pie to get married; it is hard as concrete to get unmarried. In marriage everyone wins and shares in your joy; in divorce, everyone loses except the lawyers. They profit handsomely from your misery. Everyone else shares in it.

Avoid debt, with one exception. We all need a credit card these days, but credit-card debt is killingly expensive. The interest rate will choke you to death. Don't charge more than you can pay off at the end of the month. If you can't afford it, don't buy it. Live simply and cheaply.

Buy a house as soon as you can. Buying a house is the one exception. Borrowing money to buy a house is the only debt that makes sense. Anne's and my first house was an old pre-Revolutionary (built in 1762) grist mill. We paid $3,000 for it. Cash. It needed a lot of work—a LOT of work!—which we mostly did ourselves. We lived in that old mill for thirty-eight years and raised our four children in it. Then we sold it for half-a-million dollars. Had we rented for all those thirty-eight years, paying an average monthly rent of $1,000, we would have paid out almost $500,000 in rent. Which sounds like a better deal: thirty-eight years of renting and having nothing to show for it, or paying no rent for thirty-eight years and then walking away with $500,000?

Set your own deadlines. If your teacher tells you an assignment is due in two weeks, get it done in one week, giving yourself the extra week to revise your work and make it even better. If Princeton tells you that your college application is due by midnight, November 30, get it done and off to them by noon, November 25. Your application will be stronger because you were not anxious about missing the deadline or turning in a half-baked personal statement. A deadline is by definition a *dead*-line, a line after which your work will no longer be accepted. It you miss it, you're dead. Don't die. Procrastination is the thief of time. If you put off until tomorrow what you could have done yesterday, you will never get caught up, never be able to relax. You will be forever a slave to other people's demands, to deadlines other people set for you. If you have something that needs doing, do it today.

Read, read, read. Anne read to your parents and to you all a lot when you were young. We raised Paul, Kurt, Calloway, and Nora without benefit of a television set. We took them to the library often and gave them an unlimited book-buying budget. As a result they are all excellent readers, thinkers, and writers. Your generation has computers, videogames, and smartphones, but I urge you to walk away from those devices from time to time and snuggle down with a book—a real book with paper pages and page numbers. You'll be amazed at what you can find in a book. One of the things you will find is *you*.

Write, write, write. Writing it down gives you a chance to choose your words carefully, to revise them so they say what you really mean to say, to have a record so that you can prove that you really said them, to have something worth subpoenaing by an investigative panel, and to leave a letter like this for your grandchildren.

Walk, walk, walk. If you need to get someplace, walk there. It saves money. It builds muscles. It gives you a robust appetite. It helps your digestion. It helps the environment by conserving fossil fuels. You see more. You meet neat people. You sleep better at night. You stay trim. You appreciate more immediately the lovely world you live in. You hear the birds twitter and the waves crash. You see the mountains and the valleys and the clouds and the dogs.

Risk wisely. Take some chances. If you insist on living safely in all you do, you will wind up doing nothing. You will climb no mountains, swim no rivers, buy stocks only in blue chip companies, cower at home during the day, avoid dark alleys at night, never go barefoot, experience no adventures, celebrate no triumphs. When it comes time to tell your grandchildren about your life, you will have little to contribute except how you survived by staying at home writing checks to insurance companies. No thirty-eight years fixing an old mill. No year living on an Indian reservation. No year living in Canterbury, England. No year living in China. If you always do what is safe rather than what is interesting or exciting or risky or dangerous, you will succeed only in staying safe and being boring. Take some chances. Think of yourself as the author of a novel in which you are the main character. Create some difficulties, some challenges for your main character—that is, yourself—and then find a way out of those difficulties and challenges. Don't let your life be a yawner-novel. Make your life a page-turner-novel.

Honor your body. Stay away from substances known to be harmful or addictive: tobacco, alcohol, vapors, pills, needles. It is easier to say "No" the first time than to say "No more" after the stuff hooks you.

Sail west, fail west. Inventors will tell you that the road to success is paved with many failures. Inventors will tell you how much they have learned from their failures. Inventors will tell you that hidden in every failure is a key to future success. Remember this: if there is no risk of failure in what you undertake, then it makes no sense to undertake it. If Columbus had safely sailed east, he would have found his way to the exotic spices of India—just as everyone else did. Instead he sailed west. He failed to find the exotic spices of India, but what a magnificent failure it was! It is all right to make mistakes. Mistakes make news. Mistakes make you.

Death sentence. Imagine for a moment that you have just been to the doctor, and she has told you that you have a disease that will kill you in two years, but that you will be a hundred percent healthy for those two years until your sudden death. Given that prediction, how would you spend those last two years? If your answer is different from what you are now doing, I suggest you find a way to do with one of the next two years what you would do with both of them if the prediction were true. After all, it may be.

Tell the truth, mostly, but not always the whole truth. Some truths you have a right to keep to yourself. Sometimes the truth can do no good: "You look really awful in those yellow shorts"; "You stink!"; "I dreamed I danced with Sally again last night, only this time we were both naked "; "Mother never really liked you "; "I think the president is a lot smarter than he appears to be." It is all right to have a few secrets.

Distinguish between need and want. You need clothes for warmth, protection, and modesty. You don't need seventeen pairs of shoes or fourteen baseball hats or a low-slung sports car or a first-class seat on an airplane or a rubber ducky. You need air but not perfume. You need water but not champagne.

Find a teacher, be a teacher. Most of you will have sixteen or more years of formal schooling. In those sixteen years you will have—how many?—teachers. Maybe fifty-odd teachers. A few will be really odd. A few will be really good. A few will be really bad. Most will be adequate. One may be downright evil; avoid him or her. But one of them will be just what you need. Find that one. You have a right to one really good teacher in sixteen years of schooling. And one is all you really need. Find that one. Learn all you can from her or him. Listen, observe, imitate, thank. And vow to be, to at least one other person before you die, a teacher as important as that teacher has been to you.

Focus on others, not yourself. Good teachers say little about themselves. Rather, they quickly learn that successful teachers keep the focus on their students. Know this: People are more interested in themselves than in you. Be self-reliant and strong and energetic in pursuit of your personal goals, but don't keep talking about yourself. You'll learn more if you talk about others or get them to talk about themselves.

Walk away from anger and angry people. Venting your anger can sometimes be healthy, but it is hell for the person being vented at. I've noticed that the angriest people rarely blame themselves for causing the situations that anger them. They almost always blame someone else, usually someone near and dear. Try to steer clear of anger. Try to steer clear of angry people.

Get over the awful things you've done. In the last chapter I mentioned the terrible day I asked my neighbor and best buddy Marcus Nicholas if he wanted to help me cut a limb off a tree. He said sure. An hour later he was knocked off the ladder by the falling limb and bumped his head on a rock. A couple of hours later he died. I was devastated with grief and guilt. But it was too late to redo that awful morning with awe-ful mourning. I had his widow to look after and a family to raise, and I had to get on with both those endeavors. Some things you can't replay and can't fix. You can only move on. So move on.

Don't whine, don't envy. It is easy to see negatives, to whine about your lot in life, your poverty, your looks, your prospects, your parents, your health. Before you indulge such thoughts, make a list of all the amazingly lucky things in your life: the country you were born in, the parents you were born to, the gene pool you spring from, the house you grew up in, the schools you attended, the brothers, sisters, cousins, and friends you grew up among, the grinding poverty you never felt, the grandmother you grew up knowing, the air you breathe, the shower you get clean in, the fact that you are not starving to death, the fact that when you turn the spigot water comes out—and you can drink it! How amazing is that?

Drink water. Sodas rot your teeth and make you fat and diabetic. Alcohol clouds your judgment and makes you do stupid things, and then even stupider things. The earth's supply of fresh, drinkable water is being depleted rapidly. Drink it. Hoard some gallons of water in your basement in preparation for an attack or an earthquake. Don't waste water by watering your lawn or your golf course. Yellow gold is gold. Black gold is oil. Crystal gold is water. Only one is worth cherishing.

Don't fight dying. Do your best to stay healthy, but when your time comes—and it will—try to remember that it is undignified to fight the inevitable. Live life to the hilt, but when it is time to step off the trail so as not to impede the progress of those behind you, step off boldly, confidently, and cheerfully. Life is like a ride on an escalator. When you get to the top, step off bravely. To refuse to do so is to clog the exit and to impede the ability of those behind you on the moving stairway. Say "thanks" and "bon voyage" to a few of those behind you on the trail, then stride aside to see what adventures lie behind that pretty bush off there to the risky right.

Ignore the silly babbling of old men. Nod and smile politely when they give you advice, then go forth boldly and confidently to learn for yourself the lessons that life has to teach you. Enjoy what lies ahead. Being alive is a ton of fun. You have made it so for me!

Thanks. Bon voyage. Go in peace.

I love you.

Peter G. Beidler
(also known as [aka] "Grandpa, "Grannypete," "Gramps,"
"Pop-Pop," and "Hey")

Endnote: The End of the Trail

Don't be depressed.
I need this rest
To feel refreshed.
I have been blessed.

I love my life.
I love my wife.
Two sons that shine
Two daughters fine,
And grandkids nine.

It's sure been fun.
Now sets the sun.
My work is done.
My tale is spun.

It's time to go
And join the flow.
No need to pine,
I'm doing fine.
The victory's mine.
Now go and dine!

Works Cited

NOTE: The numbers in square brackets refer to the reference numbers that I assign to the book in my *Parkinson Pete's Bookshelves: Reviews of Eighty-Nine Books about Parkinson's Disease* (Seattle: Coffeetown Press, 2018).

Bailey, Melissa. "Some seniors considering option of 'rational suicide'." *Seattle Times*, June 24, 2019, p. A4. Originally published by the *Washington Post*.

Cason, Terry. *Power Over Parkinson's: How to Live Your Best Life Even after Your Parkinson's Disease Diagnosis.* San Bernardino, California, 2016 [B34].

Claflin, Vikki. *Shake, Rattle, and Roll with It: Living and Laughing with Parkinson's*, 2nd edn, Mill Creek Publishing, 2016 [B35].

De León, Maria, MD. *Parkinson's Diva: A Woman's Guide to Parkinson's Disease.* Copyright Maria De León, 2015 [B29].

Fox, Michael J. *Lucky Man: A Memoir*. New York: Hyperion, 2002 [B5].

Gawande, Atul, MD. *Being Mortal: Medicine and What Matters in the End*. New York: Henry Holt, 2014.

Hallows, Jolyon E. A *Parkinson's Life and a Caregiver's Roadmap*. Burnaby, British Columbia, Canada: WCS Publishing, 2018.

Hebb, Michael. *Let's Talk about Death (Over Dinner)*. New York: De Capo Press, 2018.

Humphrey, Derek. *Final Exit: The Practicalities of Self-Deliverance and Assisted Suicide for the Dying*, 3rd edn. New York: Delta, 2002.

Isaacs, Tom. *Shake Well Before Use: A Walk around Britain's Coastline*. King's Lynn, Norfolk: Cure for Parkinson's Press, 2007 [B8].

James, Trudy, et al. "Speaking of Dying." Seattle: Heartwork, 2015 (Video: www.speakingofdying.com).

Jenkinson, Stephen. *Die Wise: A Manifesto for Sanity and Soul*. Berkeley: North Atlantic Books, 2015.

Kalanithi, Paul, MD. *When Breath Becomes Air*. New York: Random House, 2016.

Kinsley, Michael. *Old Age: A Beginner's Guide*. New York: Tim Duggan Books, 2016 [B33].

Kondracke, Morton. *Saving Milly: Love, Politics, and Parkinson's Disease*. New York: Ballantine, 2001 [B2].

Lazzarini, Alice. *Both Sides Now: A Journey from Researcher to Patient*. Copyright by Alice Lazzarini, 2014 [B22].

Lieberman, Abraham N., MD. *100 Questions and Answers about Parkinson Disease*, 2nd edn. Sudbury, Massachusetts: Jones and Bartlett Publishers, 2011 [A13].

Low, Daniel, MD. "Why won't we talk about death?" *Seattle Times*, May 18, 2019, p. A7.

McGoon, Dwight C., MD. *The Parkinson's Handbook*. New York: W. W. Norton, 1990 [B1].

Mistry, Rohinton. *Family Matters*. New York: Vintage International (Random House), 2002 [C4].

Parashos, Sotirios, A., MD, Rose Wichmann, and Todd Melby. *Navigating Life with Parkinson's Disease*, New York: Oxford University Press, 2013 [A15].

Parkinson, James. *An Essay on the Shaking Palsy*. London: Neely and Jones, 1817. Reprinted in the *Journal of Neuropsychiatry Clinical Neuroscience*, 12.2 (Spring, 2002), pp. 223–36.

The Peripatetic Pursuit of Parkinson Disease. Little Rock, Arkansas: Parkinson's Creative Collective, 2013 [B20].

Pernisco, Nick. *Parkinson's Warrior*. Seattle: Connected

Neurosciences LLC, 2019.

Rehm, Diane. *On My Own*. New York: Alfred A. Knopf, 2016 [A27].

Robb, Karl A. *A Soft Voice in a Noisy World*. Fairfax. Virginia: RobbWorks, 2012 [B19].

Shacter, Phyllis. *Choosing to Die, a Personal Story: Elective Death by Voluntarily Stopping Eating and Drinking (VSED) in the Face of Degenerative Disease*. Copyright 2017 by Phyllis Shacter.

Tisdale, Sallie. *Advice for Future Corpses: A Practical Perspective on Death and Dying*. New York: Simon and Schuster, 2018.

Woodall, Wendall. *Shuffle: A Way Forward, Whatever the Challenge*. Charlotte, North Carolina: Highway 51 Publishing, 2014 [B 24].

Zitter, Jessica Nutik, MD. *Extreme Measures: Finding a Better Path to the End of Life*. New York: Penguin Random House, 2017.

About the Author

PETER G. BEIDLER, AKA PARKINSON PETE, won all
sorts of teaching awards during his forty years of teaching
British and American literature at Lehigh University. He was
named National Professor of the Year in 1981 by the Council
for Advancement and Support of Education (CASE). About the
time he retired from Lehigh, he was diagnosed with Parkinson's
disease. An avid reader, he began collecting and reading books
about the disease. As he read, he wrote reviews of each one
to guide other readers as to their contents.These reviews he
gathered together as *Parkinson Pete's Bookshelves: Reviews
of Eighty-Nine Books about Parkinson's Disease*, published by
Coffeetown Press in early 2018.

He has published eight other books with Coffeetown Press:
*Army of the Potomac: The Civil War Letters of William Cross
Hazelton of the Eighth Illinois Cavalry Regiment, Chaucer's
Canterbury Comedies: Origins and Originality, The Collier's
Weekly Version of Henry James's Turn of the Screw, A Reader's
Companion to Salinger's Catcher in the Rye, Risk Teaching:
Reflections from Inside and Outside the Classroom, Self-
Reliance, Inc., A Student Guide to Chaucer's Middle English*,
and *Writing Matters*.

CPSIA information can be obtained
at www.ICGtesting.com
Printed in the USA
LVHW021613020620
657244LV00007B/1110